ULCE COMPREHENSIVE DIET GUIDE AND COOKBOOK

More than 130 Recipes and 200 Essential Tips for Ulcerative Colitis Patients

Monet Manbacci, Ph.D.

(Edition-1)

Copyright © 2019 by Monet Manbacci.

All Right Reserved.

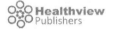

DISCLAIMER NOTICE

No part of this publication may be reproduced, distributed, or transmitted in any form or by any means, including photocopying, recording, or other electronic or mechanical methods, or by any information storage and retrieval system without the prior written permission of the publisher, except in the case of very brief quotations embodied in critical reviews and certain other noncommercial uses permitted by copyright law.

Please, consider that the information in this book is only for educational purposes. No warranties of any kind are implied or declared in this book. Readers acknowledge that the author of this book is not engaged in the rendering of medical, legal, financial, or professional advice. Hence, consult a licensed professional before applying any hints or techniques outlined in this book. By reading this notice, the readers agree that the author of this book is not responsible for any direct or indirect losses that are incurred because of the use of the information contained in this book, including but not limited to inaccuracies, omissions, and errors.

This book has been published by the Healthview Publishers. All rights reserved.

Table of Contents

Disclaimer Notice 2

Introduction 12

Chapter 1. Healthy Ulcerative Colitis Nutritional Choices 16

    Food Mis-Combination 17

    Bad Digestion 18

Chapter 2. Diet Comparisons for Ulcerative Colitis patients? 20

    Paleo Diet 20

    Modified Paleo Diet 21

    Yeast-Free Diet or Candida Free Diet 23

    Low FODMAP Diet 26

    Microbiome Diet 29

    Specific Carbohydrate Diet (SCD) 31

    Low Fiber Diet 33

    Liquid Diet for Ulcerative Colitis patients 34

    Low Residue Diet 35

Chapter 3. Comprehensive List of Recommended Foods (to Avoid & to Eat) for Ulcerative Colitis Patients 38

    Fruits 39

    Vegetables 41

    Herbs 44

    Spices 46

    Oils 47

    Animal Proteins 49

    Seafood 50

    Whole Grains 51

    Refined Grains 52

    Gluten-Free Flour Options 53

    Nuts 54

Seeds 55

Legumes 56

Sweeteners 57

Dairy Products 59

Lactose-Free Yogurt Products 60

Butter 60

Lactose-Free Milk Products 61

Cheeses 62

Sauces, Dips, and Gravies 64

Ready Foods (In General) 66

Chapter 4. How to Cook for Ulcerative Colitis patients 69

Cooking Styles/Methods 69

Food Ingredients 70

Fruits and Vegetables 70

Rice, Noodle and Pasta 71

Meat and Poultry 72

Seafood 74

Grains 74

Soy, Eggs, and Firm Tofu 76

Dairy Products 76

Spices and Herbs 77

Cheese 78

Oils 79

Sauce, Gravy, Salad Dressings 80

Drinks 81

Meals 82

Breakfast 82

Soups 83

Salads 83

Snacks 84

Desserts 85

Side Dishes 85

Chapter 5. Cooking Recipes for Ulcerative Colitis patients 87

Breakfasts 87

Gluten-Free Fluffy Pancake 87

Banana and Apple Pancakes 88

Eggs, Salmon, and Avocado 90

Baked Apple 91

Pear Oatmeal Bars 92

Avocado & Egg Breakfast Toast 94

Smoothie Bowl 96

Zucchini Bread Oatmeal 97

Breakfast fruit salad 98

Banana Split Oatmeal 100

Egg Tacos with Avocado 101

Crispy Hash Brown with Egg 102

Grilled Almond Butter Honey Banana Sandwich 104

Avocado-Cheese Bagel 105

Pineapple-Ginger Oatmeal 106

Apple Cinnamon Oatmeal 108

Appetizers 109

Turkey Potpie Soup 109

Potato-Ginger Miso Soup 111

Parsnip/Carrot Potato Soup 113

Pumpkin Soup 114

Stracciatella Soup 116

Ham and Potato Soup 118

Butternut Squash Soup 119

Chicken Noodle Soup 121

Creamy Chicken Soup 123

Seafood Chowder Soup 125

Barley/Oatmeal Soup 126

Lentil Soup 128

Homemade Vegetable Broth 130

Homemade Beef Broth 132

Russian Chicken Soup 134

Baba Ghanoush 135

Salmon Bruschetta 137

Guacamole-Like Appetizer 138

Homemade Lebanese Hummus 140

Crab Dip with Wonton Chips 142

Shrimp Salad 144

Zucchini Salad (Spiralized) 145

Olivier Salad (Chicken, Potato & Egg salad) 147

Apple-Pear Salad with A Special Vinaigrette 148

Beet, Carrot & Apple Salad 150

Butter Lettuce Salad with Honey Vinaigrette 151

Carrot-Avocado Salad 153

Classic Tuna Pasta Salad 154

Salmon Ceviche 156

Honey Mustard Chicken Salad 157

Main Courses 159

Mediterranean Chicken - Zucchini Stew 159

Lactose-Free Chicken Fettuccine Alfredo 161

Chicken with Mashed Potatoes 164

Chicken Stroganoff 166

Chicken Kebab 168

Roasted Chicken with Pomegranate Sauce 170

Puffy Chicken 172

Chicken Scaloppini 174

Chicken-Pineapple Pizza 176

Turkey Zucchini Noodles 177

Zucchini Egg Dish 179

Potato Cutlet 181

Ginger Sticky Pork 182

German Pork Schnitzel 184

Pineapple Pork 186

Balsamic-Peach Pork 188

Honey-Turmeric Pork 190

Grilled Lean Beef Kebab 192

Hungarian Goulash 194

Tomato Free Spaghetti Bolognese 196

Lamb/Beef Liver stew 198

Grilled Honey Salmon 199

Oven-based Salmon and Potato 201

Lemon Steamed Halibut with White Rice 203

Thunfisch Pizza 205

Avocado Tuna Pita 206

Trout with Orange 208

Chicken and Shrimp Teriyaki 210

Lemon Shrimp with White Rice 211

Honey Prawn Linguine 213

Desserts 215

Pineapple Cake Sundaes 215

Apple-Ginger Sundaes 216

Banana Lemon Trifle 218

Warm Apple Crumble 219

Ginger Fruit Sherbet 221

Apple Quesadillas 223

Middle-Eastern Rice Pudding 224

Gluten-Free Apple Pie 226

Pumpkin Pie 228

Fruit Dessert 229

Avocado Pear Popsicle 231

Lemon Sorbet 232

Ingredients 232

Mango Ice Cream 234

Sweet potato pie 235

White Panna Cotta 237

Cocktails and Shakes 239

Banana Milkshake 239

Cooler Drink 240

Mango-Banana Smoothie 241

Ginger Cool Drink 242

Avocado Smoothie 243

Banana-Cinnamon Smoothie 244

Peach-Mango-Banana Smoothie 245

Peach-Ginger Smoothie 246

Pomegranate-Angelica Smoothie 247

Apple-Ginger Smoothie 249

Bloody Red Drink! 250

Pineapple-Mango Smoothie 251

Cantaloupe Smoothie 252

Cantaloupe-Mix Smoothie 253

Applesauce-Avocado Smoothie 255

Pina Colada Smoothie 256

Snacks 257

Diced Fruits 257

Plain Yogurt with Poached Fruits 257

Poached Fruit Compote 257

Applesauce 259

Homemade Applesauce 259

Avocado Dip 260

Homemade Hummus 262

Tofu 264

Avocado Tofu Toast 264

Almond Butter Sandwich 265

Gluten-Free Muffins 267

Cheese Sticks 269

Avocado Tuna Toast 269

Rice Crackers 271

Gluten-Free Rice Cracker 271

Ginger Biscuits 272

Gluten-Free Ginger Biscuits 273

Zucchini Chips 274

Healthy Potato Chips 276

Drinks 277

Recommended Hot Beverages 277

Recommended Cold Beverages 281

Chapter 6. Food Preparation & Meal Planning for Ulcerative Colitis
patients 284

Eating Habits 284

Grocery Shopping 285

Cooking Tools 286

Kitchen preparation 288

Meal Planning 288

Other Tips 290

Chapter 7. Bi-weekly Cooking Plan for Ulcerative Colitis patients ... 292

Cooking Plan for Remission Periods: 292

Cooking Plan for Flare-Up Periods 295

Biweekly Cooking Plan for Ulcerative Colitis patients – Blank 298

Chapter 8. Top 200 Ulcerative Colitis Tips & Eating Patterns 301

Last Words 316

One Last Thing 318

About The Author 319

Other Books By Healthview Publishers: 320

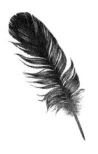

For those who Live with Ulcerative Colitis…

INTRODUCTION

Ulcerative Colitis (UC) is a type of Inflammatory Bowel Disease (IBD) that can affect colon of the GI tract. The symptoms may vary over time in their severity, and sometimes it can be excruciating and hard to tolerate, which is called flare-up periods. It can also be silent with no or few symptoms during some periods called remission. Ulcerative Colitis is a chronic non-contagious disease, which the main reason of developing it is still unknown. Research studies show the involvement of three main factors: immune system malfunction, genetics and environment. Crohn's disease is another type of IBD, that has similar symptoms to Ulcerative Colitis. However, Crohn's disease can affect the whole gastrointestinal tract (GI) from the mouth to the anus. Ulcerative Colitis can only affect the colon or the large intestine. The other difference is regarding the inflammation type. Crohn's patients typically see healthy areas between inflamed locations, but Ulcerative Colitis patients do not see healthy areas between their inflamed spots.

This book is not just a cookbook for Ulcerative Colitis patients. It gives the readers lots of information about healthy nutritional choices, food to eat or to avoid, food preparation, meal planning, and how to create biweekly cooking plans.

This book aims to primarily provide readers with necessary nutritional information about Ulcerative Colitis and then guide readers on their Ulcerative Colitis cooking and dietary plans. This book is recommended to the groups below:

1. You are an Ulcerative Colitis patient and want to know how to manage your UC diet, how to cook varieties of foods, and how to balance your meals using effective meal plans.
2. You have an Ulcerative Colitis patient in your family and want to know how to prepare Ulcerative Colitis-friendly meals or make meal plans.
3. You recently diagnosed with Ulcerative Colitis
4. Your loved one newly diagnosed with Ulcerative Colitis

If you recently diagnosed with Ulcerative Colitis or if your loved one recently diagnosed with Ulcerative Colitis, this book is an excellent source for you to take initial necessary dietary steps, learn how to cook varieties of foods for flare-up and remission periods, how to manage your disease, how to do meal planning and learn about diet tips related to the disease.

If you are an Ulcerative Colitis patient for a long period, the information in this book can also help you maintain your remission periods and balance your life with UC better than before by using recommended tips, and various cooking recipes.

This book summarizes the essential hints you need to know about this disease in plain English. Ulcerative Colitis can certainly cause issues when it comes to choosing what you eat and drink. Not only does the condition cause digestive tract inflammation and uncomfortable symptoms, but long-term consequences can even include malnutrition. To make matters more complicated, your dietary habits may worsen symptoms. While there's no cure-all diet known for Ulcerative Colitis, eating and avoiding certain foods may help prevent flare-ups. Hence, key chapters of this book focus on dietary topics such as:

- Healthy nutritional choices for UC patients
- Diet comparison for Ulcerative Colitis patients?
- Food preparation and Meal planning

Comprehensive lists of foods to avoid and foods to each for Ulcerative Colitis patients for flare-up and remission periods are presented in Chapter 3 of this book. Not so many books have provided you with such a comprehensive chapter.

The book then fully covers how to cook for Ulcerative Colitis patients following by more than 130 cooking recipes for Ulcerative Colitis patients. This chapter covers various types of recipes for breakfast, appetizers, soups, salads, snacks, main courses, desserts, and drinks. Each recipe starts with a brief explanation, preparation time, cooking time, total time, ingredients, instructions, cooking tips, UC-related tips, and nutrition facts.

The nutrition facts of the recipes in this book have been analyzed by "Verywell fit" Recipe Nutrition Calculator (Ref: https://www.verywellfit.com). The following chapters make this book unique compared with other books in the market:

- Chapter 6: gives **biweekly cooking plan samples** for flare-up and remission periods. The chapter has blank biweekly cooking plan tables for you to write your cooking plans and stick them to your fridge.
- Chapter 7: gathers the **top 200 tips for Ulcerative Colitis patients** to live healthier and happier. You can learn these pages to know more about essential

lifestyle, diet, and cooking tips for Ulcerative Colitis patients.

It has to be reminded that the recommendations, hints, and tips provided in this book have been gathered from various UC-related research studies and references from different online/offline resources. These have been found useful by the author of this book, but it does not mean that all will work for you. It should be understood that any recommendations or tips in this book can only be followed only when you take responsibility for it. Be sure that you always talk to your doctor or dietician about the recipes, steps, or hints this book recommends to make sure that they are in line with your health condition.

Chapter 1. Healthy Ulcerative Colitis Nutritional Choices

Researches show the positive effect of a healthy diet on a wide range of serious health problems. Particularly when managing chronic concerns like Ulcerative Colitis, planning a diet of foods and beverages that help minimize the flare-ups and prevent future consequences is the best way to ensure happy, comfortable and productive life now and for years to come.

Because Ulcerative Colitiscan negatively affect the colon in the digestive tract, evaluating all aspects of diet is important. Modifying diet in keeping with the information currently available will do much to inhibit unexpected bouts of serious symptoms of Ulcerative Colitis. Both the intensity and the frequency of attacks will be moderated if dietary adjustments are made. The key is eating the right foods, avoiding foods that trigger episodes and keeping quantities in check during any one meal.

Work on balancing proteins and carbohydrates in your diet, adding just a small amount of high quality, unsaturated fat. Everyone who suffers from Ulcerative Colitis has a slightly varying tolerance to different feet. Hence, consider keeping a great food diary. Note what you eat and record any reactions, positive or negative, to your choices.

Fruits and vegetables are full of water and fiber, both of which are helpful in maintaining healthy bowel movements. Occasionally particular types will cause problems, but you will be able to catch that issue with your food diary and include required nutrients, minerals, and vitamins in your diet.

Usually many people with UC should avoid dairy products. Mounting evidence leans toward following a gluten free diet as well as staying caffeine and alcohol-free. Vegetables from the Brassica family like cabbage and broccoli can also be troublesome. When selecting proteins for managing UC's symptoms emphasize sources low in saturated fats and oily fish with high levels of healthy Omega-3. Consider a high quality Omega-3 supplement if fish is hard to find or otherwise unappealing.

Experts advises eating sparingly at each meal so as not to overwhelm the digestive system of an Ulcerative Colitis sufferer. They suggest eating several well-balanced small meals each day to keep symptoms at bay.

Keep staying hydrated is also of critical importance. Not only do all the tissues of your body require proper hydration to function as intended, flushing toxins out of your system is important, especially when dealing with a disease that impacts the digestive system. Keep it simple and drink lots of water, aiming for consuming at least eight glasses per days.

Remember that changes in diet alone will not cure Ulcerative Colitis but will go along way toward reducing the symptoms and damage the condition causes. As research continues more natural ways to mitigate the disease will be uncovered. Keep abreast of these developments for optimum health.

FOOD MIS-COMBINATION

One of the things most Ulcerative Colitis sufferers hear from their doctors is to try to figure out what foods cause flare-ups, and stop eating those foods. Unfortunately, this is not a lot of help, because for many Ulcerative Colitis sufferers, any food can start the cycle of pain and misery.

The main reason that certain foods seem to worsen Ulcerative Colitis symptoms is because those foods are eaten with the wrong other foods. In other words, the foods are mis-combined. What does mis-combined mean?

Different types of foods trigger the release of different types of digestive enzymes, some acidic and others alkaline. Alone, each type of enzyme does a great job breaking down foods as nature intended. When both types of digestive enzymes are released at the same time, that is when trouble can develop.

What happens is the alkaline and acid enzymes neutralize each other and neither type of enzyme can do its job. Digestion is greatly impaired and your meal does not get broken down properly. With no working enzymes break it down, all that undigested food sits in your stomach for hours and ferments, rots, and putrefies until it is forced into the small intestine. The result is gas, heartburn, cramps, bloating, diarrhea, flatulence, you name it, with poor nutritional absorption on top of everything else.

Mis-combined foods cause misery from one end of the digestive tract to the other. Most seriously, mis-combined, poorly digested foods can get impacted or stuck in the colon, causing pain, constipation and flare-ups of diverticulitis and Ulcerative Colitis.

BAD DIGESTION

Nothing the human body does requires more energy than digestion - not exercise, not sex, nothing. So, when your stomach is working frantically, releasing all that hydrochloric acid and pepsin to try to digest poorly combined meals, you are searching either for a place to take a nap, or for a cup of coffee. Bad digestion leaves you dragging yourself around like the walking dead.

The highly acidic nature of the typical modern diet just makes matters worse. All that excess acid in the food not only contributes to heartburn and acid reflux problems, but it creates an acidic environment in your entire body. Some say that our bodies were designed to be alkaline, so a body that is acidic will also have a lowered immune system. Also, a poorly functioning immune system can keep your body from being able to fight off bacterial bugs, viruses and disease. For people prone to digestive problems, the consequences of poorly combined foods (or hard-to-digest foods) is an assault on their digestive systems and their overall health.

If you want to improve your Ulcerative Colitisor any other digestive problems, you have to eat in a way that allows your body to comfortably digest foods without excess acid. If you do so, you will find you can eat huge varieties of foods that you previously thought you could not tolerate.

The next chapter of this book compares different types of diets Ulcerative Colitis patients may want to follow and explains the best diets for Ulcerative Colitis patients.

Chapter 2. Diet Comparisons for Ulcerative Colitis patients?

There are lots of different types of diets recommended for people to have a healthy life. A typical question for an Ulcerative Colitis patient is: **which diet works best for me**? This chapter explains some of the popular diets in brief and compares them with each other to evaluate which diet works for Ulcerative Colitis patients and which does not work.

Paleo Diet

The idea of the Paleo diet is eating various foods, but do not consume processed foods at all. In other words, this diet avoids any meals with the processing cycle. Some of the foods to avoid in the Paleo Diet are:

-   Processed foods
-   Canned foods
-   GMO foods
-   Sugars: black and brown
-   Artificial sweeteners
-   Dairy products
-   Margarine
-   Sweet fruits
-   Vegetable oils
-   Foods high in Trans Fat
-   Products with High Fructose Corn Syrup (HFCS)
-   Grains
-   Legumes
-   Soft Drinks

In some dietitian's opinion, the main idea of the Paleo diet to avoid processed food is rational as processed food can produce harmful bacteria for the gut. The diet recommends eating organic fresh fruits and vegetables. In other words, you can consume anything fresh without any industrial process involved in production stages.

MODIFIED PALEO DIET

In a modified version of this diet, some foods have been added to the listed of allowing foods to use. In general, these foods are healthy foods such as:

- Gluten-Free grains
- Healthy fats such as grass-fed butter

It seems that the main problem with the Paleo diet with grains is not yeast inside grain products such as bread, but gluten, which differentiates it with the Yeast-Free diet.

Now, let us see if the Paleo diet is best for Ulcerative Colitis patients or not. Here are some advantages of the Paleo Diet for Ulcerative Colitis patients:

- Paleo diet avoids processed foods that typically, Ulcerative Colitis patients may not tolerate during flare-up periods.
- Paleo diet forbids unhealthy fatty foods that are good for Ulcerative Colitis patients, as well.
- The consumption of HFCS foods is forbidden in the Paleo diet, which is good for the health of all people, including Ulcerative Colitis patients.
- This diet avoids drinking sodas and soft drinks, which is good for Ulcerative Colitis patients, as well.

- Paleo diet avoids using legumes that can produce gas and make bloating in some Ulcerative Colitis patients.
- Paleo avoids taking dairy products and avoids/limits taking products with gluten. Some Ulcerative Colitis patients need to avoid lactose or gluten, as well.
- In general, Paleo is a protein-based diet, which is suitable for many Ulcerative Colitis patients, as well.

However, some of the issues following the Paleo diet can provide for Ulcerative Colitis patients are as below:

- Paleo diet limits taking fresh fruits that are great for Ulcerative Colitis patients, such as a banana. Moreover, some fruits/vegetables not recommended for Ulcerative Colitis patients, such as broccoli and tomatoes, but they are allowed to eat on the Paleo diet.
- Hence, the Paleo diet allows for consuming various types of vegetables that cannot be used by Ulcerative Colitis patients, especially during flare-ups. Ulcerative Colitis patients need to cook some vegetables before using them.
- Paleo diet allows you to consume fresh nuts. However, some Ulcerative Colitis patients cannot consume nuts in their normal shape.
- Many Ulcerative Colitis patients can tolerate lactose and gluten. Hence, it seems unnecessary for them to avoid consuming them. Patients need to make their own decision if these products are against their general health or not. If the answer is yes, they can follow this part of the Paleo and not use dairy or gluten products. It is highly recommended for UC patients to avoid lactose and gluten during flares.

- Paleo diet avoids using healthy grains for Ulcerative Colitis patients, such as white rice.
- Some Ulcerative Colitis patients in moderation can consume some legumes such as almonds and soybeans, although these are forbidden in the Paleo diet.

In brief, the Paleo diet cannot be an excellent diet for people with Ulcerative Colitis as it allows some not recommended foods for Ulcerative Colitis patients. It also forbids some foods that can be used by Ulcerative Colitis patients (or even recommended for them to consume).

However, some of the Paleo features such as avoid consuming processed food, not taking fast foods and sodas, not taking specific legumes, avoid using artificial sweeteners can help Ulcerative Colitis patients as well. Some other Paleo features, such as avoid consuming gluten or dairy products, depend on the health condition of Ulcerative Colitis patients. If a patient is lactose intolerant, she/he cannot consume lactose. If a patient is gluten intolerant, she/he cannot use gluten products.

YEAST-FREE DIET OR CANDIDA FREE DIET

This diet is designed based on a theory that the main reason for having a leaky gut is the overgrowth of bad bacteria in your gut. Some of the supporters of this diet are saying that bad bacteria in the gut need to be substituted by good bacteria, which can be done by not consuming yeast and add functional fermentation foods to your diet to increase the number of good bacteria in your gut. Hence, a yeast-free diet or Candida free diet forbids anything with yeast and processed foods. Some foods to avoid in the yeast-free diet are:

- Processed foods
- Anything with yeast such as bread
- Glutens
- Starchy vegetables
- High sugar fruits
- Added sugars
- Alcohols
- Limit caffeine intakes

In brief, a yeast-free diet recommends consuming the followings:

- Eat fermented foods such as yogurt, sauerkraut, apple cider vinegar, miso, etc.
- Gut-healing foods and supplements such as cabbage juice and bone broth
- Consume organic proteins, non-starchy vegetables, and non-sweet fruits
- Increase water intake

Now, let us see if the yeast-free diet is right for Ulcerative Colitis patients or not. Here are some advantages of the Paleo Diet for Ulcerative Colitis patients:

- Eating well-tolerated fermented foods might be suitable for Ulcerative Colitis patients.
- In general, consuming probiotic supplements are best for Ulcerative Colitis patients, as well.
- Some recommended gut-healing foods such as bone broth are great for Ulcerative Colitis patients as well.
- Limiting alcohol and caffeine is an excellent strategy for Ulcerative Colitis patients, as well.

However, some of the issues following the yeast-diet can provide for Ulcerative Colitis patients are as below:

-   Yeast-free diet limits taking fresh fruits/vegetables that are great for Ulcerative Colitis patients, such as carrots. Moreover, some fruits/vegetables are not recommended for Ulcerative Colitis patients, such as blackberry, broccoli, lettuce, and tomatoes, but they are allowed to eat in the Yeast-free diet.
-   The yeast-free diet allows consuming various types of non-starchy vegetables such as cauliflower and cabbage that cannot be used by Ulcerative Colitis patients, especially during flare-ups. Ulcerative Colitis patients need to cook some vegetables before using them.
-   The yeast-free diet avoids consuming moldy nuts and seeds. However, some Ulcerative Colitis patients can have nuts in moderation.
-   Many Ulcerative Colitis patients can tolerate gluten. Hence, it seems unnecessary for them to avoid consuming them. Patients need to make their own decision if these products are against their general health or not. If the answer is yes, they can follow the yeast-free and not use gluten products.
-   The Candida-free diet avoids consuming kinds of seafood, such as canned tuna. However, tuna is recommended for many of Ulcerative Colitis patients.

In brief, the yeast-free diet cannot be an excellent diet for people with Ulcerative Colitis as it allows some foods that are not recommended for Ulcerative Colitis patients, and it forbids some foods that can be taken by Ulcerative Colitis patients or even recommended for them to consume.

However, some of the yeast-free features such as avoid consuming processed food, taking probiotics and fermented foods, limit taking caffeine and alcohol, and avoid using artificial sweeteners can help Ulcerative Colitis patients as well. Another yeast-free diet feature avoids consuming gluten (depending on your health condition). If a person is gluten intolerant, she/he cannot use gluten products.

Low FODMAP Diet

This diet is mostly for people with Irritable Bowel Syndrome (IBS). This diet avoids FODMAP sugars (Fermentable Oligo-, Di-, Mono-saccharides, and Polyols). Some researchers believe that some foods with FODMAP sugars cannot be well-digested by IBS people. As such, they introduce an elimination stage and a reintroduction stage for a low FODMAP diet. In the elimination stage, IBS patients should avoid all foods that contain FODMAP sugars. After elimination, each food will be reintroduced again to the body to check if the gut can tolerate it well or not.

Some of the main avoided foods in the low FODMAP diet are:

- Foods with fructose such as sweet fruits, HFCS, sweeteners, honey, concentrated fruits, fruit juices, and dried fruits.
- Lactose products such as cow milk and cheeses with lactose
- Foods with fructans such as wheat cereals and pasta, broccoli, cauliflower, watermelon, etc.
- Foods containing polyols such as peach, pear, plum, corn, mushroom, and artificial sweeteners

- Foods with galactans, such as red beans, lentils, and chickpeas

Now, let us see if the low FODMAP diet is fine for Ulcerative Colitis patients or not. Here are some advantages of the low FODMAP diet for Ulcerative Colitis patients:

- Avoids some sugary foods that typically, Ulcerative Colitis patients may not tolerate during flare-up periods.
- Low FODMAP diet forbids unhealthy fatty foods, which is suitable for Ulcerative Colitis patients, as well.
- Consumption of foods with HFCS is forbidden in the low FODMAP diet, which is good for the health of all people, including Ulcerative Colitis patients.
- This diet avoids drinking sodas and soft drinks, which also recommends for Ulcerative Colitis patients.
- The low FODMAP diet avoids using beans that can produce gas and make bloating in some Ulcerative Colitis patients.
- The low FODMAP avoids taking products with lactose and avoids/limits taking products with gluten. Some Ulcerative Colitis patients need to avoid lactose or gluten, as well.

However, some of the issues the low FODMAP diet can provide for Ulcerative Colitis patients are:

- The low FODMAP diet limits taking fresh fruits that are great for Ulcerative Colitis patients, such as watermelon and pear. Moreover, some fruits are not recommended for Ulcerative Colitis patients, such as berries, but they are allowed to eat on the FODMAP diet.

- The low FODMAP diet allows for consuming various types of vegetables that cannot be used by Ulcerative Colitis patients, especially during flare-ups. Ulcerative Colitis patients need to cook some vegetables before using them.
- Many Ulcerative Colitis patients can tolerate lactose and gluten. Hence, it seems unnecessary for them to avoid consuming them. Patients need to make their own decision if these products are against their general health or not. If the answer is yes, they can follow the diet and not use dairy or gluten products.
- The low FODMAP diet allows using white sugar and forbids honey. However, this may need work for Ulcerative Colitis patients.

In brief, the low FODMAP diet cannot be an excellent diet for people with Ulcerative Colitis as it allows some foods that are not recommended for Ulcerative Colitis patients, and it forbids some foods that can be taken by Ulcerative Colitis patients or even recommended for them to consume.

However, some of the low FODMAP features such as avoid consuming hard-to-digest vegetables, not taking fast foods and sodas, not taking specific legumes, and avoid using artificial sweeteners can definitely help Ulcerative Colitis patients as well. Some other low FODMAP features, such as avoid consuming gluten or dairy products, depend on the health condition of Ulcerative Colitis patients. If a patient is lactose intolerant, she/he cannot consume lactose. If a patient is gluten intolerant, she/he cannot use gluten products.

MICROBIOME DIET

The main idea behind creating this diet is to provide a program to improve gut health. The Microbiome Diet has three phases. In phase-1, four steps need to take into account:

- Remove any toxins, chemicals, hormones, steroids, antibiotics, and pesticides from the body by not consuming such foods
- Repair the gut with healthy foods and supplements
- Replace the gut with edible herbs, fruits, spices, and supplements
- Reintroduce right foods to the gut to repopulate healthy gut bacteria

In brief, the foods that should be avoided during the 1st phase are grains, legumes, starchy vegetables, starchy fruits, egg, dairy products, fried foods, artificial sweeteners, fish, meat, and processed foods.

The second phase provides a type of meal plan to boost metabolism to grow healthy bacteria. The last stage is lifetime tune-up by maintaining good gut bacteria growth with a healthy meal plan.

Now, let us see if the Microbiome diet is excellent for Ulcerative Colitis patients or not. Here are some advantages of the Microbiome diet for Ulcerative Colitis patients:

- Avoids food with antibiotics and steroids are suitable for the general health of Ulcerative Colitis patients.
- The microbiome diet forbids unhealthy fatty foods, which is suitable for Ulcerative Colitis patients, as well.

- Consuming processed food is forbidden in the Microbiome diet, which is good for the health of all people, including Ulcerative Colitis patients.
- This diet avoids drinking sodas, which is recommended for Ulcerative Colitis patients, as well.
- The Microbiome diet avoids using overly sugary foods, which is suitable for Ulcerative Colitis patients, as well.
- The Microbiome diet avoids taking products with gluten. Some Ulcerative Colitis patients need to avoid gluten as well.

However, some of the issues following the Microbiome diet can provide for Ulcerative Colitis patients are as below:

- The Microbiome diet limits taking foods that are great for Ulcerative Colitis patients, such as oatmeal and egg. Moreover, some fruits are not recommended for Ulcerative Colitis patients, such as berries and cherries, but they are allowed to eat fruits in the Microbiome diet.
- The Microbiome diet allows for consuming various types of vegetables that cannot be used by Ulcerative Colitis patients, especially during flare-ups. Ulcerative Colitis patients need to cook some vegetables before using them.
- Many Ulcerative Colitis patients can tolerate gluten. Hence, it seems unnecessary for them to avoid consuming them. Patients need to make their own decision if these products are against their general health or not. If the answer is yes, they can follow the diet and not use gluten products.

- The Microbiome diet allows using some nuts such as walnuts. However, some Ulcerative Colitis patients should limit or avoid taking nuts and seeds.

In brief, the Microbiome diet cannot be an excellent diet for people with Ulcerative Colitis as it allows some foods that are not recommended for Ulcerative Colitis patients, and it forbids some foods that can be taken by Ulcerative Colitis patients or even recommended for them to consume.

However, some of the Microbiome features such as avoid consuming processed food, not taking fast foods, sugary foods and sodas, not taking refined oils, and avoid using artificial sweeteners can help Ulcerative Colitis patients as well. Some other Microbiome features, such as avoid consuming gluten, depend on the health condition of Ulcerative Colitis patients. If a patient is gluten intolerant, she/he cannot use gluten products.

SPECIFIC CARBOHYDRATE DIET (SCD)

This diet aims to limit poorly digestible carbohydrates, which may lead to reduce gas, diarrhea, and cramping. Some of the foods to avoid in the SCD diet are:

- Processed meats
- Starchy vegetables such as potatoes and yam
- Added sugars
- Coffees
- Artificial sweeteners
- Additives such as HFCS, corn starch, etc.
- Canned fruits
- Dried fruits with added sugar
- Grains: rice, pasta, bread, etc.
- Dairy products

- Oil sprays

Now, let us see if the SCD diet is suitable for Ulcerative Colitis patients or not. Here are some advantages of the SCD diet for Ulcerative Colitis patients:

- Avoids food with HFCS is good for the general health of Ulcerative Colitis patients.
- The SCD diet forbids unhealthy fatty foods, which is suitable for Ulcerative Colitis patients, as well.
- Consuming processed meat is forbidden in the SCD diet, which is good for the health of all people, including Ulcerative Colitis patients.
- The SCD diet avoids using added sugar foods, which is suitable for some Ulcerative Colitis patients, as well.
- The SCD diet avoids taking products with dairy. Some Ulcerative Colitis patients need to avoid lactose, as well.

However, some of the issues following the SCD diet can provide for Ulcerative Colitis patients are as below:

- The SCD diet limits taking foods that are great for Ulcerative Colitis patients, such as oatmeal, potatoes, and rice. Moreover, some fruits are not recommended for Ulcerative Colitis patients, such as berries and cherries, but they are allowed to eat fruits on the SCD diet.
- The SCD diet allows for consuming various types of vegetables that cannot be used by Ulcerative Colitis patients, especially during flare-ups such as chickpeas. Ulcerative Colitis patients need to cook some vegetables before using them.

- Many Ulcerative Colitis patients can tolerate grains. Hence, it seems unnecessary for them to avoid consuming them. Patients need to make their own decision if these products are against their general health or not. If the answer is yes, they can follow the diet and not use so many grain products with gluten.
- The SCD diet allows using dried fruits and vegetables such as tomatoes that are not good for Ulcerative Colitis patients, especially during flare-up periods.

In brief, the SCD diet cannot be an excellent diet for people with Ulcerative Colitis as it allows some foods that are not recommended for Ulcerative Colitis patients, and it forbids some foods that can be taken by Ulcerative Colitis patients or even recommended for them to consume.

However, some of the SCD features such as avoid consuming processed food, not taking fast foods, not taking added sugars, and avoid additives such as HFCS can help Ulcerative Colitis patients as well. Some other SCD features, such as avoid consuming lactose, depend on the health condition of Ulcerative Colitis patients. If a patient is lactose intolerant, she/he cannot use dairy products with lactose.

LOW FIBER DIET

This diet is suitable for people who cannot have fiber for any reason. Doctors may recommend this diet to some of Ulcerative Colitis patients who had colon surgical procedures. The main idea is to avoid eating foods high in fiber. This diet is one of the diets that are good to follow if you have UC, diverticulitis, or ulcerative colitis. Some foods to avoid in the low fiber diet are:

- Whole-grain foods such as brown rice & oat

- Anything whole wheat such as whole wheat pasta or bread
- Foods with seeds and nuts
- Corns and popcorns
- Berry fruits
- Lentils
- Granolas
- Dried fruits
- Foods that produce gas such as broccoli and cauliflower (not raw, not cooked)
- Raw fruits (exceptions: melon, banana, and skin removed peach)

As explained, this diet is recommended for Ulcerative Colitis patients who had surgeries. Other Ulcerative Colitis patients can also follow this diet if they are in a flare-up.

LIQUID DIET FOR ULCERATIVE COLITIS PATIENTS

Your doctor may ask you following a liquid diet in specific circumstances temporarily such as:

- Very hard flare-up
- After a surgical procedure
- Blockages or strictures in the large intestine

The main idea is to avoid solid foods for a while to give rest to the gut and quicken the healing process. You should be under the supervision of a doctor or a nutritionist to make sure that you receive the right nutrients while taking this diet. Here are some of the tips when you need to take a liquid diet:

- Consume bone broth, chicken broth, and vegetable broth a lot.

- Fresh fruit juices do not have much fiber. You can have fresh fruit juices from recommended fruits.
- It is recommended to purchase a juicer or a blender. Having a juicer is recommended as it can break down the fibers from your fruit/vegetable juices.
- Cook soups and then blend them with a blender.
- You can combine fruit juices with vegetable juices, as well.
- Drink plenty of water.
- Some patients can use Gatorade. Ask your doctor about it.
- Remove any pulp from the juices before drinking them.

LOW RESIDUE DIET

A low residue diet is another diet that can be asked to follow if you are an Ulcerative Colitis patient. This diet can add residue to the stool and can lessen diarrhea and abdominal pains and cramps, which is suitable for people with UC who had surgeries in their large intestines.

Some of the foods to avoid in a low residue diet include, but not limited to:

- Nuts (including almond and coconut) and seeds
- Raw fruits such as berries
- Dried fruits
- Some fruit juices such as prune juice
- Raw and leafy vegetables
- Jams and marmalades
- Whole grains
- Pickles
- Strong seasonings such as pepper, chili, and garlic

- Legumes
- Popcorns and corns
- Hard to digest cheeses
- Fried and processed meats
- Fried eggs
- Fried foods and fried pastries

The recommended foods to allow and foods to avoid in this book are well-matched with a low-residue diet. Generally speaking, some diets recommended for Ulcerative Colitis patients are high in proteins and high calorie, as some Ulcerative Colitis patients need to have a faster healing process. Your doctors may ask you to combine the low fiber diet with the low residue diet. In this case, you need to follow both diets at the same time. The next chapters of this book can help you write your diet plan based on the foods that you can well-tolerated during remission and flare-ups. Table 1 summarizes the result of different diet comparison for Ulcerative Colitis patients.

Table 1. Diet Comparison for Ulcerative Colitis patients

Diet Name:	Description:	Good choice for Ulcerative Colitis patients?	Counterexample:
Paleo	Do not eat processed foods	No	You can eat tomato and broccoli in the Paleo diet. Many Ulcerative Colitis patients cannot eat them during a flare-up.
Modified Paleo	Same as Paleo but allows gluten-free grains and some other healthy foods	No	You cannot eat oatmeal in modified Paleo. Many of Ulcerative Colitis patients can eat oatmeal.
Low FODMAP	Avoid consuming FODMAP sugars.	No	Many fruits, such as apple or pear, are forbidden, but not for

	Great for IBS patients		Ulcerative Colitis patients.
Yeast-Free	Avoid anything with yeast. May heal Candida Overgrowth	No	Bread and many fruit juices are forbidden, but not for many of Ulcerative Colitis patients.
Microbiome	A 4 R's meal plan to eliminate trigger foods, metabolic boost meal plan, and lifetime tune up	No	Eggs cannot be eaten in the Microbiome diet, but many Ulcerative Colitis patients can eat eggs as a great source of protein.
Specific Carbohydrate Diet (SCD)	Limits poorly digestible carbohydrates	No	White rice and potatoes are forbidden, but not for Ulcerative Colitis patients.
Low-Fiber	Consume low-fiber foods as liquids	Yes. For patients with surgeries	-
Liquid Diet	Consume foods in liquid format only.	Yes. For patients with severe flares, surgeries or strictures	-
Low Residue	Avoid seeds, nuts, raw fruits, etc.	Yes. For patients with surgeries or large intestine strictures	-
Your Own	An Ulcerative Colitis patient needs to find a specific diet for herself/himself	Yes (The best for each Ulcerative Colitis patient)	-

Chapter 3. Comprehensive List of Recommended Foods (to Avoid & to Eat) for Ulcerative Colitis Patients

This chapter provides comprehensive lists of foods to eat and foods to avoid for Ulcerative Colitis patients for flare-up and remission periods. To cover a variety of foods from "safe foods to eat," to "triggering foods to avoid," five different colors are defined as indicators as follows:

G	The food is safe to consume.
B	It is recommended to consume this food in moderation.
Y	Each Ulcerative Colitis patient needs to check this food to see if the food is tolerable or not.
O	It is recommended not to consume or limit taking this food.
R	Avoid consuming this food.

Different food categories are investigated, and the tips related to flare-up and remission periods are explained in this chapter.

As such, you can see one of these five colors in front of each food in food category lists, which can help you decide whether to go with that food item or not.

Remember, it does not mean that the foods highlighted in blue can be consumed without tolerance checking. It means that according to research studies, experiences of Ulcerative Colitis patients, or expert recommendations, they are more likely to be safe and non-triggering. Always test your tolerance regarding foods in blue color.

On the contrary, it does not mean that the foods highlighted in orange cannot be consumed. It means that according to research studies, experiences of Ulcerative Colitis patients, or expert recommendations, they are more likely to trigger. Always test your tolerance regarding foods in orange color, have your research and, if you decide to consume, have them in little amounts or use them in moderation. Table 2 to Table 22 present foods to eat and to avoid for flare-up and remission periods.

FRUITS

During Flares

1. In many cases (except not allowed fruits in red or orange), poached, skin and core-removed fruits can be well-tolerated.
2. Make sure you do not consume poached fruits, or compotes high in sugar during flares.
3. Do not forget to eat fruits in blue color in moderation during flares.
4. Check if a fruit increases diarrhea during flare-up periods or not. If yes, avoid using it.
5. Check if the fruit is high in fiber or not. Avoid consuming it if it has high insoluble fiber inside.
6. Check if the fruit is easy to digest or not. If it is hard to digest, avoid eating it during flares.
7. Check if the fruit can help dehydration or not. Consider other factors when you choose a fruit to eat during flares.

8. Check if a fruit has anti-inflammatory properties or not. Consider other factors when you chose a fruit to eat during flares.
9. Avoid fruits with non-removable seeds during flares such as berries.

During Remissions

1. You can consume fruits shown in green color during flare-ups, but it is recommended to peel off and remove cores of fruits during the remission period as well.
2. Most fruits can be well-tolerated during remission periods.
3. Remember to eat fruits in "blue color" in moderation.
4. Be aware of consuming orange or red fruits during remission periods.

Table 2. List of fruits to eat and to avoid for Ulcerative Colitis patients

Fruits:	Flare-up	Remission
Apple	B	G
Apricots	O	B
Avocado	G	G
Banana Ripe	Y	G
Banana	B	G
Banana Unripe	B	G
Barberries	O	Y
Blackberries	O	Y
Blueberries	O	Y
Cantaloupe	G	G
Carambola/Starfruit	G	G
Cherries	R	O
Clementine	O	G
Coconut	O	B
Cranberries	O	B
Date	O	G
Dragonfruit	O	G
Durian	O	B
Feijoa	R	B
Figs	R	B

Goji berries	R	Y
Gooseberries	R	Y
Grapefruit	O	G
Grapes	O	Y
Guava	R	B
Honeydew Melon	G	G
Jackfruit	Y	G
Java-Plum	Y	G
Jujube Fruit	Y	G
Kiwifruit	O	B
Kumquat	O	G
Lemon	G	G
Lime	G	G
Longan	Y	G
Loquat	O	G
Lychee	Y	G
Mandarin	O	G
Mango	B	G
Mangosteen	Y	G
Mulberries	O	O
Nectarine	B	G
Olives	G	G
Orange	O	G
Papaya	G	G
Passion Fruit	O	B
Peaches	B	G
Pear	O	G
Persimmon	O	B
Pineapple	B	G
Plums	O	Y
Pomegranate	B	G
Prunes	R	O
Quince	O	B
Raisins	R	O
Raspberries	O	O
Rhubarb	R	O
Strawberries	R	O
Tamarind	B	G
Tangerine	O	G
Watermelon	G	G

VEGETABLES

During Flares

1. In many cases (except not allowed vegetables in red), boiled or steamed, skin-removed vegetables can be well-tolerated.
2. Make sure you do not stir fry vegetables during flare-up periods.
3. Eat vegetables in blue in moderation during flares.
4. Check if a vegetable increases diarrhea during flare-up periods. If yes, avoid eating it.
5. Check if a vegetable is high in insoluble fiber or not. If yes, avoid consuming it or boil it.
6. Check if a vegetable is easy to digest or not. If it is hard to digest, avoid eating it during flares.
7. Check if a vegetable has anti-inflammatory properties or not. Consider other factors when you chose a vegetable to eat during flares.

During Remissions

1. It is recommended to consume tolerable vegetables (raw or boiled) during the remission period.
2. Many vegetables can be well-tolerated during remission periods (highlighted in green).
3. Remember to eat vegetables in blue in moderation.
4. Try to consume vegetables with fiber, folic acid, vitamin A, C, E, and K, calcium, and other required nutrients for Ulcerative Colitis patients.

Table 3. List of vegetables to eat and to avoid for Ulcerative Colitis patients

Vegetables:	Flare-up	Remission (Raw)	Remission (Boiled)
Amaranth Leaves	R	O	Y
Alfalfa	R	O	Y
Arrowroot	R	O	Y
Artichoke	R	O	Y
Arugula	R	O	Y
Asparagus	R	Y	B

Bamboo Shoots	R	O	Y
Beans, Green	O	B	B
Beets	R	Y	B
Belgian Endive	R	O	Y
Bok Choy	R	O	Y
Broccoli	R	R	O
Brussel Sprouts	R	O	Y
Cabbage, Green	R	R	O
Cabbage, Red	R	R	O
Carrot	G	G	G
Cauliflower	R	R	O
Celery	Y	O	Y
Celery Root	R	O	Y
Chicory	R	O	Y
Collards	R	O	Y
Corn	R	R	R
Cucumber	B	B	G
Edamame	R	Y	B
Eggplant	O	Y	B
Fennel	R	O	Y
Ginger Root	B	B	G
Horseradish	R	O	Y
Jalapeño	R	R	O
Kale	R	O	Y
Kohlrabi	O	Y	B
Leeks	R	O	Y
Lettuce, Butter	B	B	G
Lettuce, Iceberg	R	O	O
Lettuce, Leaf	R	O	O
Lettuce, Romaine	R	O	O
Mushrooms	O	O	Y
Mustard	Y	B	G
Okra	R	O	Y
Onion, Red	R	R	O
Onions	R	R	O
Parsnip	R	O	Y
Peas, Green	R	O	Y
Pepper, Green	R	O	O
Pepper, Red	B	O	O
Potato, Red	B	G	G
Potato, White	Y	B	G
Potato, Yellow	G	G	G
Pumpkin	G	G	G
Radishes	R	O	Y
Shallots	R	R	Y

Spaghetti Squash	G	B	B
Spinach	O	Y	B
Squash, Butternut	G	B	B
Sugar Snap Peas	R	O	Y
Sweet Potato	Y	Y	B
Swiss Chard	R	O	Y
Tomatillo	R	O	Y
Tomato	R	O	Y
Turnip	R	O	Y
Yam Root	Y	O	Y
Zucchini	B	G	G

HERBS

During Flares

1. Remember to eat herbs in blue color in moderation during flares.
2. It is fine to boil or steam herbs and consume during flares.
3. Check if an herb is easy to digest or not. If it is hard to digest, avoid eating it during flares.
4. Check if an herb has anti-inflammatory properties or not. Consider other factors when you chose an herb to consume during flares.

During Remissions

1. Many herbs can be well-tolerated during remission periods.
2. Use more herbs with anti-inflammatory properties and rich in nutrients and vitamins required for Ulcerative Colitis patients during remission periods.

Table 4. List of herbs to eat and to avoid for Ulcerative Colitis patients

Herbs:	Flare-up	Remission
Aloe Vera	R	G
Angelica	Y	G
Basil	Y	G

Bay	Y	G
Bee Balm	R	B
Calendula	Y	G
Caraway	R	B
Catnip	R	B
Cayenne	R	R
Chamomile	Y	G
Chives	R	B
Cilantro	R	B
Cinnamon	G	G
Coriander	R	B
Dill	R	B
Fennel	R	B
Garlic	R	O
Geraniums	R	B
Ginger	G	G
Ginseng	B	G
Hibiscus	R	B
Horseradish	R	B
Laurel	R	B
Lavender	Y	B
Lemon Balm	Y	B
Lemongrass	O	B
Lemon Zest	Y	G
Licorice Root	O	B
Marjoram	R	B
Milk Thistle	R	B
Mint	Y	G
Nettle	Y	G
Oregano	O	G
Parsley	O	B
Peppermint	Y	G
Rosemary	Y	G
Saffron	Y	G
Sage	R	B
Salvia	R	B
Savory	R	B
Sweet bay	R	B
Sweet cicely	R	B
Sweetgrass	R	B
Tarragon	R	B
Thyme	Y	G
Tulsi / Holy Basil	Y	G
Turmeric	G	G
Yarrow	R	B

SPICES

During Flares

1. Do not forget to consume spices in blue color in moderation during flares.
2. Check if a spice is hot and spicy. If yes, avoid consuming it during flares.
3. Check if a spice has anti-inflammatory properties or not. Consider other factors when you chose a spice to use during flares.

During Remissions

1. Many spices can be well-tolerated during remission periods.
2. Use more herbs with anti-inflammatory properties and rich in nutrients and vitamins required for Ulcerative Colitis patients during remission periods.

Table 5. List of spices to eat and to avoid for Ulcerative Colitis patients

Spices:	Flare-up	Remission
Angelica	Y	G
Bay leaf	Y	G
Basil	Y	G
Bergamot	Y	G
Black cumin	O	G
Black mustard	Y	B
Black pepper	R	Y
Burnet	Y	G
Caraway	R	B
Cardamom	Y	G
Catnip	R	B
Cayenne pepper	R	R
Chicory	O	G
Chili pepper	R	R
Chives	R	B
Cicely	O	G
Cilantro	R	B

Cinnamon	G	G
Clove	R	B
Coriander	R	B
Cumin	Y	G
Curry	R	B
Dill	R	B
Fennel	R	B
Fenugreek	R	B
Ginger	G	G
Holy basil	Y	B
Horseradish	R	B
Lavender	Y	B
Lemon balm	Y	B
Lemongrass	O	B
Licorice	O	B
Marjoram	R	B
Nutmeg	R	B
Oregano	Y	G
Paprika	R	O
Parsley	Y	B
Peppermint	Y	G
Poppyseed	R	B
Rosemary	Y	G
Saffron	Y	G
Sage	R	B
Salt	G	G
Sesame	R	O
Spearmint	Y	G
Sumac	Y	B
Tarragon	R	B
Thyme	Y	G
Turmeric	G	G
Vanilla	Y	G
White mustard	Y	G

OILS

During Flares

1. It is highly recommended to avoid consuming lots of oil during flare-up periods. Most meals should be boiled or cooked without consuming oils.

2. A safe option for cooking during flares is using extra virgin olive oil in moderation.
3. Avocado and fish oils are also other safe options.

During Remissions

1. Ulcerative Colitis patients can consume most cooking oils during remission periods. However, it is recommended to avoid consuming palm and corn oils.
2. Always try to consume high-quality organic oils.
3. Remember that the best options are extra virgin olive oil and avocado oil.
4. Check your tolerance if you want to cook your meal with any of the oils shown in yellow in the table below.

Table 6. List of oils to eat and to avoid for Ulcerative Colitis patients

Cooking Oils/Fats	Flare-up	Remission
Butter	R	Y
Olive Oil	B	G
Extra Virgin Olive Oil	G	G
Coconut Oil	B	G
Animal Fats	R	O
Palm Oil	R	O
Avocado Oil	G	G
Fish Oil	B	G
Flax Oil	R	Y
Canola Oil	O	Y
Nut Oils and Peanut Oil	**Flare-up**	**Remission**
Peanut oil	R	Y
Macadamia nut oil	Y	G
Seed and Vegetable Oils	**Flare-up**	**Remission**
Soybean oil	R	Y
Corn oil	R	O
Cottonseed oil	R	Y
Rapeseed oil	R	Y
Sunflower oil	R	Y
Sesame oil	R	Y
Grapeseed oil	R	B

Safflower oil	R	Y
Rice bran oil	R	Y

ANIMAL PROTEINS

During Flares

1. Avoid eating skins and fat cuts.
2. Avoid eating cold cuts.
3. Avoid eating spicy cold cuts.
4. Avoid eating hard to digest meats.
5. Avoid eating animal proteins with the skin.
6. Eat animal proteins shown in blue color in moderation.
7. Use lean or extra lean cuts for red meat and pork if you can tolerate them during flares.
8. The ostrich is an excellent source of protein to try during flares.
9. Poaching and boiling eggs are the best methods of making eggs during flare-up periods.

During Remissions

1. Remove skins of poultries and other animal proteins before consumption.
2. Stick to lean and extra lean cuts during remission periods as well.
3. Remember to eat animal proteins in blue in moderation.
4. Try to limit red meats in your meal plan.
5. Put high amounts of animal proteins in your weekly meal plan.
6. Avoid consuming fatty parts of meat, chicken, and pork during remission periods, as well.

Table 7. List of animal proteins to eat and to avoid for Ulcerative Colitis patients

Animal Proteins	Flare-up	Remission
Red Meat:		
Beef	R	Y
Bison	R	Y
Goat leans	R	Y
Lamb	R	Y
Moose	R	Y
Ostrich	B	G
Venison	R	Y
Veal	R	Y
Kangaroo	R	Y
Lean/Extra Lean Red Meat	B	G
Eggs:		
Chicken eggs	B	G
Quail eggs	B	G
Poultry:		
Chicken	G	G
Turkey	G	G
Duck	G	G
Goose	G	G
Pork:		
Pork	R	O
Ham	R	O
Bacon	R	O
Pork Lean	B	G
Pork Tenderloin	B	G
Other:		
Sausage	R	O
Pepperoni	R	O
Salami	R	O

SEAFOOD

1. Seafood is an excellent source of healthy fatty acids for Ulcerative Colitis patients.
2. Always (during flares or remissions) put seafood in your weekly meal plan.
3. Remember to consume seafood shown in blue color in moderation during flare-up periods.

4. It is recommended to avoid consuming scallops or caviars during flare-up periods.

Table 8. List of seafood to eat and to avoid for Ulcerative Colitis patients

Seafood	Flare-up	Remission
Tuna	G	G
Salmon	G	G
Trout	G	G
Bluefish	G	G
Catfish	G	G
Halibut	G	G
Clams	B	G
Oyster	B	G
Mussels	B	G
Crab	G	G
Lobster	G	G
Shrimps	G	G
Prawns	G	G
Scallop	O	B
Caviar	O	B

WHOLE GRAINS

1. It is recommended not to consume whole grains during flare-up periods at all. Oatmeal can be checked and then, consumed during flares.
2. During remission, consuming whole grains depend on the health condition of an Ulcerative Colitis patient. If an Ulcerative Colitis patient has a complication such as strictures, or a part of large intestine surgically removed, she/he needs to avoid whole grains.
3. It is also recommended for other Ulcerative Colitis patients to avoid consuming whole grains in the remission period as well. Oatmeal family and quinoa are excluded from this rule. They can be consumed in moderation if they can be tolerated well.

Table 9. List of whole grains to eat and to avoid for Ulcerative Colitis patients

Whole Grains	Flare-up	Remission
Amaranth	R	O
Barley	O	Y
Brown Rice	R	O
Brown Rice Bread	R	O
Brown Rice Tortilla	R	O
Buckwheat	R	O
Bulgur (Cracked Wheat)	R	O
Farro / Emmer	R	O
Flaxseed	R	O
Grano	R	O
Kamut / Khorasan	R	Y
Millet	R	O
Oats	O	Y
Oat Bread	O	Y
Oat Cereal	O	Y
Oatmeal	Y	B
Popcorn	R	R
Whole Wheat Cereal Flakes	R	O
Muesli	R	O
Rolled Oats	R	B
Quinoa	R	Y
Rye	R	O
Sorghum	R	O
Spelt	R	O
Teff	R	O
Triticale	R	O
Whole Grain Barley	R	O
Wheat Berries	R	O
Whole Grain Cornmeal	R	O
Whole Rye	R	O
Whole Wheat Bread	R	O
Whole Wheat Couscous	R	O
Whole Wheat Crackers	R	O
Whole Wheat Pasta	R	O
Whole Wheat Pita Bread	R	O
Whole Wheat Sandwich Buns And Rolls	R	O
Whole Wheat Tortillas	R	O
Wild Rice	R	O

REFINED GRAINS

1. Some of the white refined grains such as white rice, macaroni, and pasta can be well-tolerated during flare-up periods. Hence, consider them in your flare-up meal plan.
2. Most of the white grains can be well-tolerated during remission periods.
3. It is recommended not to consume grain products with corn.
4. It is recommended to consume organic, non-GMO grains.

Table 10. List of refined grains to eat and to avoid for Ulcerative Colitis patients

Refined Grains	Flare-up	Remission
Cornbread	R	O
Corn Tortillas	R	O
Couscous	O	Y
Crackers	O	G
Flour Tortillas	O	B
Noodles	B	G
Spaghetti	B	G
Macaroni	B	G
Pitas	B	G
Pretzels	Y	Y
Ready-To-Eat Breakfast Cereals	O	Y
White Bread	B	G
White Sandwich Buns and Rolls	B	G
White Rice	G	G

GLUTEN-FREE FLOUR OPTIONS

1. Many gluten-free flours may not be tolerated well during remission periods. It is recommended to avoid consuming them if it is possible.
2. On the contrary, many gluten-free flour options can be well-tolerated during remission periods, but it is

recommended to consume gluten-free flours without whole grains.

3. Flours from nuts should be well-grounded.
4. Do not consume flours with high non-soluble fibers during flares.

Table 11. Gluten-free flours to eat and to avoid for Ulcerative Colitis patients

Gluten-Free Flours	Flare-up	Remission
Almond Flour	Y	G
Buckwheat Flour	O	Y
Sorghum Flour	O	Y
Amaranth Flour	O	Y
Teff Flour	O	Y
Arrowroot Flour	Y	B
Brown Rice Flour	R	O
Oat Flour	Y	B
Corn Flour	R	O
Chickpea Flour	R	Y
Coconut Flour	O	Y
Tapioca Flour	O	B
Cassava Flour	O	B
Tigernut Flour	R	B

NUTS

During Flares

1. It is highly recommended to avoid consuming raw nuts during flare-up periods.

During Remissions

1. Remission2: Some of Ulcerative Colitis patients without having intestine complications can consume limited amounts of nuts. It is recommended for this group to check their tolerance regarding each type of nuts they want to eat.

2. Remission1: It is highly recommended for Ulcerative Colitis patients with large intestine complications such as strictures, or any other complications from the large intestine surgeries, to avoid consuming nuts during flares and remission periods.
3. Some nuts such as almond can be used in moderation in other formats such as smoothened almond butter or almond milk and if they can be well-tolerated.
4. Make sure the almond butter or other nut butter you want to consume is smooth.
5. You can also make stews with well-ground nuts if you can tolerate them.

Table 12. List of nuts to eat and to avoid: Remission1 patients with colon complications, Remission2: typical Ulcerative Colitis patients

Nuts	Flare-up	Remission1	Remission2
Almond	R	O	B
Black Walnut	R	O	Y
Brazil Nut	R	O	Y
Butternut	R	O	Y
Candlenut	R	O	Y
Cashew	R	O	B
Chestnuts	R	O	Y
Hazelnut	R	O	Y
Hickory Nut	R	O	Y
Macadamia	R	O	Y
Oak Acorns	R	O	Y
Pecan	R	O	Y
Persian Walnuts	R	O	Y
Pine Nut	R	O	Y
Pistachio	R	O	Y
Walnut	R	O	Y
White Nut	R	O	Y

SEEDS

During Flares

1. It is highly recommended to avoid consuming seeds during flare-up periods.

During Remissions

1. Remission2: Some of Ulcerative Colitis patients without having intestine complications can consume limited amounts of seeds. It is recommended for this group to check their tolerance regarding each type of seeds they want to eat.
2. Remission1: It is highly recommended for Ulcerative Colitis patients with large intestine complications such as strictures, or any other complications from the large intestine surgeries, to avoid consuming seeds during flares and remission periods.

Table 13. List of seeds to eat and to avoid: Remission1 patients with colon complications, Remission2: typical Ulcerative Colitis patients

Seeds	Flare-up	Remission1	Remission2
Chia seeds	R	O	Y
Flaxseed	R	O	Y
Hemp seeds	R	O	Y
Poppyseed	R	O	Y
Pumpkin seeds	R	O	Y
Sesame seed	R	O	Y
Safflower	R	O	Y
Sunflower	R	O	Y

LEGUMES

1. Avoid consuming legumes during flares.
1. It is recommended not to consume legumes highlighted in orange color even during remission.
2. Check your tolerance level when you want to consume legumes shown in yellow color.
3. You may consume green peas in moderation during remission periods.

Table 14. List of legumes to eat and to avoid for Ulcerative Colitis patients

Legumes	Flare-up	Remission
Adzuki beans	R	O
Black beans	R	O
Soybeans	R	Y
Anasazi beans	R	O
Fava beans	R	Y
Chickpeas	R	Y
Kidney beans	R	O
Lima beans	R	O
Peanut	R	O
Green peas	R	B
Snow peas	R	Y
Snap peas	R	Y
Split peas	R	O
Black-eyed peas	R	O
Yellow lentils	R	O
Orange lentils	R	O
Green lentils	R	O
Brown lentils	R	O
Black lentils	R	O

SWEETENERS

During Flares

1. It is highly recommended to avoid consuming artificial sweeteners during flare-up periods.
2. White sugar needs to be significantly limited during flare-up periods.
3. Patients need to check their tolerance for sweeteners such as honey or maple syrup.
4. It seems that Stevia can be well-tolerated. However, use it in moderation during flare-up periods.

During Remissions

1. It is recommended to avoid consuming artificial sweeteners, even during remission periods.

2. It is recommended to consume natural sugars or plant-based sweeteners during remission periods such as stevia (instead of white processed sugar).
3. Honey, maple syrup, molasses, and stevia seem to be some promising options for white processed sugar. Make sure you can tolerate them well.

Table 15. List of sweeteners for Ulcerative Colitis patients

Sweeteners	Flare-up	Remission	Notes:
Acesulfame K	R	O	Artificial Sweetener
Agave Syrup	Y	Y	Modified Sugar
Aspartame	R	O	Artificial Sweetener
Brown Sugar	R	Y	Sugar
Cane Juice	R	Y	Sugar Extract
Caramel	R	O	Modified Sugar
Coconut Sugar	R	B	Sugar Extract
Corn Sugar (HFCS)	R	R	Modified Sugar
Corn Sweetener (HFCS)	R	R	Modified Sugar
Corn Syrup (HFCS)	R	R	Modified Sugar
Curcumin	R	B	Natural Sweetener
Dextrose	R	O	Sugar
Erythritol	R	Y	Sugar Alcohol
Fructose Glucose Syrup (HFCS)	R	R	Modified Sugar
Glucitol (Sorbitol)	R	R	Sugar Alcohol
Glucose-Fructose Syrup (HFCS)	R	R	Modified Sugar
Golden Syrup	R	R	Modified Sugar
High Fructose Corn Syrup (HFCS)	R	R	Modified Sugar
Honey	Y	B	Natural Sugar
Mannitol	R	Y	Sugar Alcohol
Maple Syrup	Y	B	Sugar Extract
Molasses	O	B	Sugar Extract
Palm Sugar	R	O	Sugar Extract
Saccharin	R	O	Artificial Sweetener
Sorbitol	R	Y	Sugar Alcohol
Stevia, Aka Truvia or Pure Via	B	G	Natural Sweetener

Sucralose	R	O	Artificial Sweetener
White sugar (Table Sugar)	O	B	Sugar: Sucrose
Xylitol	R	Y	Sugar Alcohol

DAIRY PRODUCTS

During Flares

1. It is highly recommended to avoid consuming dairy products during flare-up periods as these products are hard to digest and can irritate your gut.

During Remissions

1. Some Ulcerative Colitis patients without lactose intolerance are typically able to consume milk, goat milk, kefir, yogurt, yogurt drinks, or other types of dairies during remission periods in moderation. This group of patients needs to avoid consuming fatty cheese even during remission. It is also recommended for this group of patients to put yogurt and kefir in their meal plan as they are excellent sources of probiotics and prebiotics, respectively.

2. UC lactose-intolerant patients need to avoid consuming dairy products with lactose, even during remission periods.

Table 16. List of dairy products to eat and to avoid for Ulcerative Colitis patients

Dairy	Flare-up	Lactose Intolerant Flare	Remission	Lactose Intolerant Remission
Milk	R	R	Y	R
Goat milk	R	O	B	O
Fermented Milk	R	R	Y	R

Kefir	O	R	G	R
Yogurt	R	R	G	R
Yogurt drinks	R	R	G	R
Cream	R	R	Y	R
Sour cream	R	R	Y	R
Fatty Cheese	R	R	O	R

LACTOSE-FREE YOGURT PRODUCTS

During Flares

1. It is highly recommended to avoid consuming yogurt products during flare-up periods.

During Remissions

1. UC lactose-intolerant patients can consume lactose-free yogurt options according to Table 18 below:

Table 17. List of lactose-free yogurt products to eat and to avoid

Lactose-Free Yogurt	Flare-up	Remission
Soy Yogurt	R	Y
Lactose-free yogurt	R	G
Almond milk yogurt	O	G
Coconut milk yogurt	O	G
Cashewgurt	R	Y
Nut yogurt (plant-based yogurt)	R	Y

BUTTER

During Flares

1. It is highly recommended to avoid consuming butter during flare-up periods.

During Remissions

1. Ulcerative Colitis patients in remission can consume butter in moderation. However, it is recommended to check your tolerance when consuming it.
2. It is also recommended not to consume salted butter.
3. The best-recommended butter option for those who can tolerate butter during remission periods is organic grass-fed butter.

Table 18. List of butter to eat and to avoid for Ulcerative Colitis patients

Butter	Flare-up	Remission
Salted Butter	R	O
Unsalted Butter	R	Y
Grass-fed Butter	R	B
Margarine	R	O

LACTOSE-FREE MILK PRODUCTS

During Flares

1. It is highly recommended to avoid consuming milk products during flare-up periods.

During Remissions

1. UC lactose-intolerant patients can consume lactose-free milk options according to the below table. They need to check alternative options to the cow milk to see if they do not have any problem consuming them.

Table 19. List of lactose-free milk products to eat and to avoid

Lactose-Free Milk	Flare-up	Remission
Almond Milk	O	G
Soy Milk	R	Y
Cashew Milk	R	Y
Rice Milk	O	G
Coconut Milk	O	G
Hemp Milk	R	Y
Pea Milk	R	Y
Oat Milk	R	G

Peanut Milk	R	O
Flax Milk	R	Y
Walnut Milk	R	Y

CHEESES

During Flares

1. It is highly recommended to avoid consuming cheese products during flare-up periods as cheeses are hard to digest foods and can irritate the gut.

During Remissions

1. Ulcerative Colitis patients who are not lactose-intolerant can consume cheese options according to the below table. They need to check cheese types and see if they can tolerate them or not.
2. For patients who are lactose intolerant, there are varieties of lactose-free options shown in blue to consume. For cheeses shown in yellow color, patients need to check if they can tolerate them or not.
3. It is recommended for patients who are not lactose intolerant to consume lactose-free cheese options as well.
4. It is recommended not to consume soft and fatty cheeses, even during remission periods.

Table 20. List of cheeses to eat and to avoid for Ulcerative Colitis patients

Hard Cheeses	Flare-up	Remission
Asiago	R	Y
Blue	R	Y
Bra	R	Y
Buffalo	R	Y
Four Herb Gouda	R	Y
Halloumi	R	Y
Jarlsberg	R	Y
Marble Cheddar	O	Y

Monterey Jack Dry	R	O
Parmesan (Parmigiano)	O	B
Parmigiano Reggiano	O	B
Pecorino	O	B
Pecorino Romano	O	B
Reggianito	O	Y
Romano	R	Y
Seriously Strong Cheddar	O	Y
Smoked Gouda	R	Y
Swiss	O	B
Yaroslavsky	R	Y
Semi-Hard Cheese		
Canadian Cheddar	R	O
Cheddar	R	O
Gouda	R	O
Monterey Jack	R	O
Provolone	R	O
Sweet Style Swiss	O	Y
Yorkshire Blue	R	O
Semi-Soft Cheese	R	O
American Cheese	R	O
Baby Swiss	R	Y
Bocconcini	R	O
Cream Havarti	R	O
Low Fat Feta	R	Y
Fresh Jack	R	O
Fromage de Montagne de Savoie	R	O
Havarti	O	Y
Monastery Cheeses	R	O
Mozzarella (Australian)	R	O
Paneer	R	O
Pasteurized Processed	R	O
Soft Cheese		
Ambert	R	O
Brie	R	O
Broccio	R	O
Broccio Demi-Affine	R	O
Cottage Cheese	R	O
Cream Cheese	R	O
Feta	R	O
Fresh Mozzarella	R	O
Fresh Ricotta	R	O
Fruit Cream Cheese	R	O
Gorgonzola	R	O

Labneh	R	O
Mascarpone	R	O
Mozzarella	R	O
Mozzarella in water	R	O
Ricotta	R	O
Goat Cheese	R	Y

SAUCES, DIPS, AND GRAVIES

During Flares

1. Avoid eating greasy and fatty sauces/gravies.
2. Avoid eating spicy sauces/gravies.
3. Avoid consuming high sugar gravies/sauces.
4. Avoid eating sauces or gravies with triggering ingredients such as onions.
5. Avoid eating hard to digest sauces/gravies.
6. Avoid eating gravies/sauces with nuts and seeds inside.
7. Remember to eat ready gravies/sauces in blue in moderation.
8. Avoid consuming sauces/gravies with milk inside during flares.

During Remissions

1. Eat gravies/sauces in green and blue in moderation.
2. Always make healthy and fresh gravies/sauces.
3. It is recommended to consume low-fat, low-sodium organic sauces.
4. Avoid spicy sauces/gravies even during remission periods.

Table 21. List of sauces to eat and to avoid for Ulcerative Colitis patients

Sauces, and Dips	Flare-up	Remission
BBQ	R	B
Apple Cider Vinegar	O	G

Sauce		
French dip	R	B
Ketchup	R	O
Mayonnaise	O	Y
Honey Garlic	R	Y
Tomato sauce	R	O
Hot sauce	R	R
Peppercorn sauce	R	R
Sour cream sauce	R	B
Mustard	Y	G
Sweet chili		
Tartar sauce	Y	B
Vinaigrette	Y	G
Wine sauce	R	O
Worcestershire sauce	R	B
Gravy	Y	B
Mushroom gravy	R	
Poutine	R	B
Thousand island	R	B
Tobasco	R	R
Onion sauce	R	O
Salsa	R	O
Applesauce	G	G
Cranberry sauce	R	Y
Mango sauce	Y	B
Strawberry sauce	R	Y
Balsamic	Y	B
White vinegar	R	B
Red vinegar	R	B
Sour grape	R	B
Béchamel sauce	Y	B
Oyster sauce	R	B
Soy sauce	Y	B
Teryaki sauce	R	B
Tzatziki	R	Y
Pesto	R	Y
Alfredo	R	B
Arrabbiata sauce	R	O
Marinara sauce	R	O
Café de Paris sauce	R	Y
Sweet chili sauce	R	R
Garlic sauce	R	O
Guacamole sauce	R	B
Mushroom sauce	R	Y
Cheez whiz	R	Y
Cheddar sauce	R	Y

READY FOODS (IN GENERAL)

During Flares

1. Avoid eating greasy and fatty foods (e.g., fast foods).
2. Avoid eating spicy foods.
3. Avoid eating foods with triggering ingredients.
4. Avoid eating hard to digest foods.
5. Avoid eating foods with lots of sugar.
6. Avoid eating processed and canned foods.
7. Avoid eating foods with high insoluble fiber.
8. Avoid eating foods with nuts and seeds inside.
9. Remember to eat ready foods shown in blue color in moderation.
10. It's better to eat low residue, low fiber foods during flares.

During Remissions

1. Always try to consume fresh and healthy foods.
2. Foods with healthy fats are also suitable for Ulcerative Colitis patients.
3. Foods rich in soluble fiber and high in protein are excellent choices during remission periods.
4. Avoid eating spicy foods and triggering foods, even during remission periods.
5. You can have meals with sugar, but make sure that the sugar has been used moderately in the meals you want to eat.

Table 22. List of ready foods for Ulcerative Colitis patients

Ready Foods	Flare-up	Remission
Applesauce	G	G
Bruschetta	R	Y

Bagels	R	B
Bisque	Y	G
Babaganoosh	R	Y
Burrito	R	O
Butter chicken	R	Y
Cake	R	B
Candy	R	B
Carne Asada	R	B
Cheeseburger	R	O
Chimichanga	R	O
Chips	R	Y
Chocolate	R	O
Chocolate Bars	R	O
Chowder	O	B
Cookies	R	B
Cupcakes	R	B
Curry	R	Y
Dumplings	Y	B
Donuts	R	Y
Enchilada	R	O
Eggrolls	Y	B
English muffins	R	B
Eel sushi	O	B
Fajita	R	B
Falafel	R	Y
Frankfurters	R	R
Fried Chicken	R	Y
Fondu	R	O
French onion soup	R	O
Gnocchi	B	G
Granola	R	B
Guacamole	R	B
Gumbo	R	Y
Grits	R	O
Graham crackers	O	B
Hamburgers	R	O
Hash browns	R	B
HFCS Products	R	O
Huenos Rancheros	R	Y
Hotdogs	R	O
Hummus	Y	G
Ice cream	R	B
Irish stew	R	Y
Indian food	R	O
Italian bread	R	Y

Kabobs	G	G
Jambalaya	R	O
Jelly/jam	R	Y
Jerky	R	Y
Lasagna	R	Y
Marshmallow	O	B
Meatballs	R	Y
Noodles	Y	Y
Charcuterie	R	O
Pizza	R	Y
Pancakes	R	Y
Quesadilla	R	Y
Quiche	R	Y
Reuben	R	Y
Rice Noodles	B	G
Sashimi	Y	G
Sorbet	Y	G
Sushi	Y	B
Tater tots	R	O
Waffles	R	B
White steamed rice	G	G
Ziti	R	Y
Zucchini Chips	B	G

Chapter 4. How to Cook for Ulcerative Colitis patients

Each Ulcerative Colitis patient is unique in terms of symptoms, complications, food intolerances, and sensitivities. That is why there is not a single UC diet for everyone. However, there are essential points that need to be taken into account when you want to cook for an Ulcerative Colitis patient:

Cooking Styles/Methods

1. The best cooking methods for Ulcerative Colitis patients are boiling, steaming, roasting, grilling, poaching, stewing, and air frying.
2. It is crucial not to fry (especially deep fry) foods during flare-up periods. If you want to fry, simmer or cook on a pan, use a small amount of extra virgin olive oil. Even you can spray it when roasting or grilling.
3. When grilling beef or poultry, make sure the inside of your meat cooked well. Always try to grill well-done.
4. You can poach fruits and boil vegetables and other meals to consume. These are the best cooking methods during flare-ups. If you are poaching fruits, make sure you use small amounts of sugar. We recommend not to use refined sugars at all. If you need a substitute for sugar, you can try stevia. Other possible options are honey, maple syrup, and agave syrup.

Remember to consume these alternatives only if you can tolerate them well.

5. Air frying is the best option if you want to have skin-removed potato chips and zucchini chips. Consume a small amount of extra virgin olive oil when you want to air fry by an air fryer.
6. Broiling is another method that can be fine with Ulcerative Colitis patients. However, Ulcerative Colitis patients should avoid eating the burned parts of broiled food.
7. In brief, the best cooking methods for an Ulcerative Colitis patient during a flare are boiling/poaching and steaming. During remission, other cooking styles can be used by consuming a moderate amount of oil. The recommended oil to use is an extra virgin olive oil (if available, buy high-quality organic one).

FOOD INGREDIENTS

FRUITS AND VEGETABLES

Fruits and vegetables contain valuable sources of nutrients that are essential for Ulcerative Colitis patients. When you have inflammation in your GI tract, you need to make sure that you eat fruits and vegetables that are very easy to digest.

1. Remember that during the remission period, Ulcerative Colitis patients can have certain raw fruits such as apple and pear. However, the skin should be removed. Making a fruit salad from these fruits is a great meal option.

2. During a severe flare-up, it is recommended to consume skin-removed poached/boiled fruits instead of raw fruits with no sugar or a tiny amount of it (if it can be tolerated).
3. During a severe flare-up, boil or steam vegetables that are easier to digest, such as asparagus and skin-removed potatoes.
4. Making a vegetable broth or stock is a great meal option for Ulcerative Colitis patients.
5. Avoid fruit and vegetable seeds.
6. Avoid juices with the pulp.
7. The best option for juicing fruits and vegetables is to use a sturdy juicer or a juicing machine. When you are juicing with such devices, you are removing the fibers of fruits and vegetables. As such, you can get vitamins, minerals, and other healthy properties of fruits and vegetables without getting their fiber. This approach is fabulous for Ulcerative Colitis patients with large intestine narrowing or strictures or any other patients who should follow a low-fiber diet.
8. The best fruit and vegetable juices for Ulcerative Colitis patients are banana, cantaloupe, melon, papaya, apple, lemon, watermelon, squash (no seeds), pumpkin, cucumber, pomegranate, carrot, celery, zucchini, and cucumber.

RICE, NOODLE AND PASTA

1. Try not to consume wild rice and brown rice. The best rice option for Ulcerative Colitis patients is white rice, such as basmati or Jasmine white rice.
2. To make an excellent rice meal, steamed white rice in a rice maker or a proper pot.

3. The best noodle option for you is Asian-style rice noodles as they are low in fiber and can be cooked so fast.
4. Another great noodle for you is egg noodles. This type of noodle is low in fiber as well, which is excellent for Ulcerative Colitis patients that need to follow a low-residue diet.
5. Alternatively, you can make zucchini noodles or spiralized zucchini using a spiralizer.
6. Cook your pasta according to its package instruction. Typically, you need to choose a proper pot and pour water on top of your pasta to cover all pasta. After boiling water, cook pasta in the boiling water for about 10 minutes. You can add salt and extra virgin olive oil to the boiling water to taste. Use them in moderation.
7. If you are not a gluten-intolerant Ulcerative Colitis patient, you can cook most of the regular pasta with gluten, but remember to use whole wheat or whole grain pasta in moderation.
8. If you are a gluten-intolerant Ulcerative Colitis patient, you can have gluten-free pasta with white rice flour or soy. You can have other types of gluten-free pasta such as quinoa or brown rice in moderation and check if you can tolerate them.
9. Alternatively, you can make spaghetti squash to have a delicious vegetarian spaghetti.

MEAT AND POULTRY

Animal proteins contain various types of vitamins and minerals, such as vitamin-B, E, zinc, magnesium, and iron. They also have amino acids that are essential for Ulcerative Colitis patients. That is why Ulcerative Colitis patients need to eat varieties of animal proteins. Moreover, Ulcerative Colitis patients need to take more protein during flare-up periods to increase the time of recovery from inflammation.

1. Do not use processed meats at all. Consuming meats that have been salted, fermented, smoked, or canned is not recommended. Avoid consuming cold-cuts and sausage products.
2. Reduce the amount of red meat you eat every week.
3. When in remission, you can have extra lean or lean red meat in moderation. Choose low-fat or no-fat cuts.
4. During a flare-up, you need to limit your red meat intake. Just use no-fat well-cooked extra lean (or lean) part or avoid consuming red meat if you are experiencing a severe flare.
5. Do not stir fry meat and poultry when you are in a flare. Cook them well in boiling water.
6. Avoid consuming fatty parts of any meat.
7. Ostrich meat without fat is one of the best red meat options for Ulcerative Colitis patients. The ostrich meat has a similar taste of beef meat, but with lower fat and cholesterol. Moreover, it is rich in protein, iron, and calcium that are fantastic for Ulcerative Colitis patients.
8. Do not eat spicy or fatty meat products such as salami and pepperoni during flare-up periods.
9. You can cook chicken/turkey breasts, legs, and thighs. Make sure the skins are removed. It is not recommended to eat chicken wings during a flare.
10. Limit the usage of pork. Use low-fat (or no fat) extra lean (or lean) part of pork meat.
11. Avoid eating bacon during flares. Limit eating it during remission, as well.

SEAFOOD

Seafood is another excellent source of protein, amino acids, and healthy fats. Oily fish contain healthful fats, including omega-3 fatty acids. This combat inflammation and may help reduce the risk of heart disease and certain cancers. Health experts often recommend eating at least two servings of oily fish per week. These can include trout, salmon, mackerel, herring, tuna, and sardines.

1. To keep fat levels as low as possible, grill the fish or bake them with small amounts of extra virgin olive oil. It is the best way to cook the fish, for easy digestion.
2. Tuna is another excellent seafood that Ulcerative Colitis patient can consume. You can make a delicious sandwich with tuna, avocado, and lemon juice. It is not recommended to eat raw sashimi such as tuna sashimi, especially if you are not sure about the place you purchased them, as you will be more vulnerable to diseases such as salmonella.
3. Well-cooked shrimps, prawns, and crabs can also be consumed in remission and flare periods.

GRAINS

Grains are excellent sources of fiber, vitamin-B, iron, and other healthy nutrients such as magnesium and selenium. In general, grains contain three components: germ, bran, and endosperm. Whole grains have all three components, but refined grains have a process of removing the germ and bran to have a smooth texture. During this process, some iron and B-vitamin can be removed from the grain. As such, some recommend consuming whole grain products during remission if you can tolerate and if you are entirely sure that you do not have any UC complications such as stricture in your large intestine. Otherwise, use refined grains.

1. Refined grains have less fermentable fiber than whole grains, so they pass more quickly through the digestive tract. They tend to be easier on the gut and less likely to cause inflammation.
2. Examples of refined grains include: white bread, white rice, pasta, plain crackers, pancakes, waffles, and rice snacks.
3. All-purpose white flour is an excellent option for cooking and baking. Alternatively, almond flour is another superb option for Ulcerative Colitis patients, especially for those who are gluten intolerant.
4. Ready-to-eat cereals that are low in fiber are also a good option. Also, fortified refined grains contain added essential nutrients, such as as vitamins and minerals. So, a person should look for fortified products. Many breads, for example, are fortified with iodine and folate. Manufacturers also tend to fortify ready-to-eat cereals with vitamins A, C, and D, thiamine, iron, and folate.
5. Remember that gluten-intolerant patients need to avoid gluten and alternatively consume non-triggering gluten-free products.
6. The oatmeal made from quick or rolled oats is a type of refined grain, with slightly less fiber than steel-cut oats. Manufacturers produce oats by removing the hulls. When experiencing a flare-up, it is best to avoid foods containing insoluble fiber, which can worsen symptoms of diarrhea. Oatmeal contains a soluble fiber called beta-glucan. It can help ease diarrhea by absorbing water in the intestines, forming a gel, slowing digestion, and adding bulk to stool.

7. Try adding oats to smoothies that contain peeled, low-fiber fruits. Breaking down food in a blender makes digestion easier. However, if you see that you cannot tolerate oatmeal well during a severe flare-up, avoid consuming it.

Soy, Eggs, and Firm Tofu

1. Soy, eggs, and tofu are great sources of lean protein. Also, egg yolks contain high amounts of vitamin D, and people with Ulcerative Colitis are often deficient in vitamin D and A.
2. In addition to lean protein, soy and tofu contain bioactive peptides, and some research suggests that these have antioxidant and anti-inflammatory properties, which may help manage UC.
3. Do not eat fried eggs or scrambled eggs during a flare-up. Alternatively, hard-boil eggs.
4. When you are in a flare, bake tofu instead of stir-frying it.

Dairy Products

1. Many yogurts contain probiotics, which are healthful bacteria that may help reduce inflammation in the gut.
2. Dairy products are rich in calcium, and manufacturers may fortify them with vitamins D and C. Many, however, contain lactose, a type of sugar, and some doctors recommend eliminating lactose from the diet. The number of dairy servings per day may depend upon the individual dietary needs of a person with Crohn's. As explained, some people with the condition find dairy products worsen their

symptoms. If not the case, a person can eat two servings or less of the following options:
- Cheese
- Cottage cheese
- Milk
- Yogurt with live active cultures

3. Lactose-intolerant patients should avoid any forms of lactose in their cooking. It is also recommended for Ulcerative Colitis patients that are not lactose intolerant to limit consuming dairy products while in flare-up as generally, dairy products are hard to be digested. Suggested alternatives are:
- Almond milk
- Coconut milk
- Oat milk
- Soy milk
- Rice milk

4. Some Ulcerative Colitis patients may not tolerate coconut milk well as it might be hard for them to digest it during flare-up periods.

SPICES AND HERBS

1- Certain spices can be used in your cooking. Turmeric, ginger, and cinnamon are great spices for UC meals as they have anti-inflammation and anti-microbial properties.
2- Salt can also be consumed. As a general health recommendation, use it in moderation.
3- Black pepper can only be used during remission periods in moderation.
4- Other hot spicy peppers such as cayenne or red pepper are not recommended.

5- Use garlic powder in moderation only if you can tolerate it.
6- Try not to use onion powder as well.
7- It is recommended to grate ginger instead of mincing it.
8- Other recommended herbs that can be used in moderation are: thyme, oregano, and saffron
9- Lemon zest can be used during remission in moderation.
10- Some studies show anti-inflammatory properties of ginseng, as well. You may want to use it in moderation if you can tolerate it well.
11- Use other common herbs such as basil, cilantro, rosemary, Angelica, and parsley in moderation if you can tolerate. Try not to consume during a severe flare-up or use a small number of cooked versions.

CHEESE

1- If you can tolerate lactose, you can consume low-fat cheeses such as feta and cheddar during remission in moderation.
2- It is recommended to limit your cheese intake when you are experiencing a flare-up. It does not matter if you are lactose intolerant or not.
3- If you are lactose-intolerant, you still can have a variety of cheese to consume. Many of Ulcerative Colitis patients with lactose intolerance can tolerate cheese with less than 0.5-gram lactose per serving in their meals. Some of the safe cheese to consume for lactose intolerant patients are:
   - Lactose-free Swiss
   - Hard grating cheeses such as Parmigiano-Reggiano and Pecorino

- Aged cheddar
- Muenster
- Aged Brie or Camembert

The abovementioned cheeses typically have less than 2% lactose in their servings, which can be tolerated by most lactose-intolerant patients. Some other cheeses with more percentage of lactose are listed below. These cheeses can also be safe (if taken in moderation) for some lactose-intolerant patients. Always check your intolerance level before consuming these cheeses:

- Havarti
- Normal Parmesan
- Provolone
- Gouda
- Blue
- Mild cheddar
- Normal Swiss

Some cheeses to avoid are soft, mozzarellas, fetas, ricottas, and cottages.

Some lactose-intolerant patients can tolerate goat cheeses better. You can check if you can tolerate goat cheese or not.

OILS

1- The best oil recommended for Ulcerative Colitis patient is extra virgin olive oil.
2- Avoid consuming butter during flare-ups. Use butter in a minimal amount during remission. The best butter to choose is grass-fed butter.
3- Avocado oil is another recommended oil to use for cooking.

4- Coconut oil might be used in moderation (but not recommended).

5- Safflower oil, grapeseed oil, sunflower oil, vegetable oil, and soybean oil are other oils that can be used in moderation. They are excellent sources of Omega-6, which is great for the correct inflammatory response in Ulcerative Colitis patients.

SAUCE, GRAVY, SALAD DRESSINGS

Here are some of the essential tips for using sauce, gravy, and salad dressings:

- Do not use hot spicy sauces, gravies, or salad dressings.
- Mayonnaise can be used in moderation in remissions only. Try to make or purchase low-fat low-sodium organic types.
- Some of Ulcerative Colitis patients cannot tolerate tomato-based products such as Ketchup, tomato sauce, and tomato paste. Check your tolerance level for these types of sauces before consuming them. Moreover, use them in moderation.
- Mustard: is fine in general. Use it in moderation during remission and flare-ups.
- Sour cream: can be used in moderation, but check your tolerance before consuming it.
- Smooth sauces and salad dressings are fine in general. Always try to check your tolerance first, and if you are okay, use them in moderation.
- Gravies: low-sodium low-fat gravies from beef and poultry are generally fine to consume in moderation.

- Soy sauce is fine in general. Always try to check your tolerance first, and if you are okay, use it in moderation.
- Balsamic vinegar is fine in general. Always try to check your tolerance first, and if you are okay, use it in moderation.
- White vinegar is fine in general. Always try to check your tolerance first, and if you are okay, use it in moderation.
- Red/White wines: avoid using wine in sauces or dressings.
- Tahini: is fine in general. Always try to check your tolerance first, and if you are okay, use it in moderation.
- Barbecue (BBQ) sauce: has a high acidity level in it. Check your tolerance first, and if you are okay, use it in moderation.
- Sauces/gravies with garlic or onion: are not recommended. Use garlic-based sauces or gravies in a minimal portion only if you can tolerate it.
- Honey and maple syrup are fine in general. Always try to check your tolerance first, and if you are okay, use them in moderation.

DRINKS

Drink options are fully explained in Chapter-10 of this book. In general, Ulcerative Colitis patients should avoid sodas, sparkling water, and fizzy beverages. Caffeine should be avoided during a flare-up and limit having caffeinated drinks during remission periods. Some herbal teas such as peppermint and green tea are great alternatives for caffeinated beverages.

MEALS

BREAKFAST

Breakfast is an essential meal for Ulcerative Colitis patients. Typically, the breakfast of Ulcerative Colitis patients should be rich in proteins and soluble fibers. Soluble fibers are easier to digest as they can absorb water and become like gels during the digestion process. Some prefer to consume foods with more carbohydrates in the morning, and some who are more concern about their weight gain want to consume foods with fewer carbohydrates for their breakfast. If you're going to have more carbs, you can consume sweet fruits that are good for Ulcerative Colitis patients more. Some of the great breakfast options for Ulcerative Colitis patients are:

- Decaffeinated hot drinks (coffee, tea, etc.)
- Eggs: Boiled eggs are recommended. However, scrambled eggs can be used in moderation during remission.
- Oatmeal: you can combine oatmeal with cinnamon, honey (If you can tolerate), applesauce, or skin-removed cubed apples to have a very delicious oatmeal breakfast.
- Banana oatmeal
- Almond butter (smoothened) sandwich
- Avocado sandwich
- Yogurt and cow milk if you can tolerate and not in a flare.
- Preferably use lactose-free yogurt with skin-removed raw or poached fruits such as papaya, pear, apple, banana during remission.

SOUPS

Soup is one of the great meals an Ulcerative Colitis patient can have during a day. Perfectly blended soups are very easy to digest and are great for patients who should have a liquid diet or Bland diet, and for patients with complications such as large intestine strictures. Soups can be more in your meal plan during flare-up periods if you can tolerate. Some of the most exceptional soups for Ulcerative Colitis patients are:

- Blended bone broth, beef broth, chicken broth, and vegetable broth
- Blended or mashed potato soup (skin-removed)
- Pumpkin soup
- Butternut squash soup
- Chicken noodle soup
- Chicken and white rice soup
- Oatmeal soup

SALADS

Salad is a great meal for most people. You can mix different types of foods with different high nutrients, vitamins, and minerals together in a salad. However, making a salad could be a challenging task for Ulcerative Colitis patients, as many typical salad ingredients cannot be well-tolerated by the Ulcerative Colitis patients. There are lots of different salads for Ulcerative Colitis patients. This book provides you with delicious salad recipes in Chapter-10. Some of the fantastic salad options and salad ingredients for Ulcerative Colitis patients include but not limited to:

- Skin-removed cucumber and carrot are great salad ingredients for Ulcerative Colitis patients.

- Fruit salad can be made from certain fruits Ulcerative Colitis patients can tolerate well.
- Many of Ulcerative Colitis patients think that they cannot eat salads with lettuce anymore. However, many of Ulcerative Colitis patients can tolerate Butter lettuce (or called Bibb lettuce) as this type of lettuce has softer leaves that can be digested easier than other types of lettuces. Try butter lettuce in moderation and check if you can tolerate it or not.
- Zucchini, potato, pasta, and chicken are other great ingredients for having a delicious salad.
- Other salad ingredients such as beets or herbs such as spinach, parsley, and basil might be used in moderation if you can tolerate them. Some Ulcerative Colitis patients cannot tolerate vegetables that contain histamine, such as spinach. Always check your tolerance and adjust your diet and meals based on that.

SNACKS

Snacks can play a crucial role in the meal plan of Ulcerative Colitis patients. Ulcerative Colitis patients need to eat smaller portions five or six times during a day. Hence, a full, healthy snack that cannot trigger the disease can be beneficial for Ulcerative Colitis patients. Here are some of the snack options for Ulcerative Colitis patients:

- Hummus
- Applesauce
- Avocado sandwich
- Gluten-free snacks
- Fruits (poached or compote)
- Rice crackers

- Oatmeal
- Zucchini chips
- Lactose-free milk, such as almond milk
- Cheese sticks (low-fat, lactose-free options)

Avoid consuming chocolates as snacks, especially if you are experiencing a flare-up.

DESSERTS

Dessert can also be an excellent meal portion for Ulcerative Colitis patients to soothe their gut. Here are some of the dessert options for Ulcerative Colitis patients:

- Ice creams made with allowed fruits: lactose intolerant patients need to use lactose-free ice creams or sorbets
- Sorbet from allowing fruits
- Shakes made with allowed fruits: lactose intolerant patients need to use lactose-free milk
- Trifle with banana and lemon
- Gluten-free cakes
- Applesauce
- Fruit compote or bowl made with allowed fruits

SIDE DISHES

Each meal can have its well-matched side dishes. Some of the side dish options for Ulcerative Colitis patients include, but not limited to:

- Roasted or boiled potatoes (skin removed)
- Mashed potatoes (recommendations: use olive oil instead of butter and lactose-free milk instead of cow milk if you are lactose-intolerant)

- Boiled vegetables such as spinach (if you can tolerate)
- Zucchini as chips, raw or roasted (skin removed)
- Cooked, raw or glazed carrots
- Mushroom: Check your tolerance first and then consume in moderation if you are fine. If not, you may use shiitake mushroom alternatively.
- Beets: are generally fine. Check your intolerance first and use it in moderation if you can tolerate it.
- Green beans are generally fine. Check your intolerance first and use it in moderation if you can tolerate it.
- Avocado: mashed or cubed
- Lemon or lime wedges
- Well-cooked asparagus or fennel
- Recommendation: try not to use tomatoes, caramelized onion, roasted garlic, raw broccoli, raw cauliflower, and corn.
- Sauerkraut can be consumed in moderation during remissions. You need to avoid consuming it during flares.
- Pickles: check your tolerance first and then consume in moderation if you are fine. Avoid using them during flares.

The next chapter of this book gives excellent cooking recipes for Ulcerative Colitis patients.

CHAPTER 5. COOKING RECIPES FOR ULCERATIVE COLITIS PATIENTS

This chapter provides you with more than 130 fantastic delicious cooking recipes for Ulcerative Colitis patients. It consists of various recipes to cook, serve, and enjoy, such as breakfasts, soups, salads, appetizers, main courses for lunch and dinner, desserts, drinks, and snacks.

Each cooking recipe starts with a brief introduction, preparation time, cooking time, total time, serving size, ingredients, instructions, cooking tips, UC-related tips, and nutrition facts. It has to be noted that the nutrition facts of the recipes in this book have been analyzed by "Verywell fit" Recipe Nutrition Calculator.

BREAKFASTS

GLUTEN-FREE FLUFFY PANCAKE

A great gluten-free pancake for those who cannot tolerate gluten. You can make this great pancake if you are lactose-intolerant, as well. Just remember to use lactose-free milk instead of kefir.

- Prep Time: 5 minutes
- Cook Time: 10 minutes
- Total Time: 15 minutes
- Serving: 4

Ingredients:

- 2 organic, free-range eggs
- 2 cups white rice flour or almond flour

- 2 cups kefir or (lactose-free milk with one tablespoon lemon juice)
- 1 teaspoon lime juice
- 1.5 tablespoon baking powder
- Salt to taste

Instructions

1. In a medium bowl, mix and whisk all ingredients.
2. Heat a large pan with extra virgin olive oil and cook both sides of pancakes until golden over medium heat.
3. Enjoy!

Cooking Tips:

- You can use maple syrup or honey with your pancakes if you can tolerate it.

UC-related Tips:

- Use lactose-free milk if you are lactose intolerant.

Nutrition Facts

Servings: 4

Amount per serving

Calories	402
	% Daily Value*
Total Fat 7.3g	9%
Saturated Fat 3.5g	17%
Cholesterol 97mg	32%
Sodium 132mg	6%
Total Carbohydrate 71.2g	26%
Dietary Fiber 3.4g	12%
Total Sugars 6.3g	
Protein 11.5g	
Vitamin D 8mcg	39%
Calcium 20mg	2%
Iron 1mg	4%
Potassium 93mg	2%

BANANA AND APPLE PANCAKES

Another yummy lactose-free, gluten-free pancake for those with IBD and IBS.

- Prep Time: 5 minutes
- Cook Time: 10 minutes
- Total Time: 15 minutes
- Serving: 2

Ingredients

- 1 apple, skin-removed
- 3 bananas, cubed
- 4 medium-sized organic, free-range eggs
- 2 cups almond flour
- 1 tablespoon extra virgin olive oil
- Honey or maple syrup (optional)

Instructions

1. In a medium bowl, mash and whisk apple, bananas, and eggs.
2. Heat a large pan with high-quality extra virgin olive oil, flatten your pancake and cook both sides until golden over medium heat.
3. Serve with honey if you can tolerate it. Enjoy!

Cooking Tips:

- You can use maple syrup or honey with your pancakes if you can tolerate it.
- Use 2 cups of white rice flour if you want to have another taste of a delicious pancake.

Nutrition Facts

Servings: 2

Amount per serving

Calories   **401**

	% Daily Value*
Total Fat 16.5g	21%
Saturated Fat 3.9g	20%
Cholesterol 327mg	109%
Sodium 126mg	5%
Total Carbohydrate 56.5g	21%
Dietary Fiber 7.3g	26%
Total Sugars 33.9g	
Protein 13.3g	
Vitamin D 31mcg	154%
Calcium 56mg	4%
Iron 3mg	14%
Potassium 871mg	19%

EGGS, SALMON, AND AVOCADO

This breakfast contains a great source of healthy fats and protein. A smooth, fast, and delicious breakfast recipe to cook!

- Prep Time: 5 minutes
- Cook Time: 10 minutes
- Total Time: 15 minutes
- Serving: 2

Ingredients:

- 2 scrambled eggs
- 2 oz salmon, cooked or canned
- 1 avocado
- 1 teaspoon extra virgin olive oil

Instructions

1. Heat a large pan with high-quality extra virgin olive oil, and scramble your eggs over medium heat.
2. Mix your scramble with avocado cubes and small salmon pieces. Enjoy!

<u>Cooking Tips:</u>

- You can also mash your avocado instead of cubing it.

<u>UC-related Tips:</u>

- Use boiled salmon and eggs if you are experiencing a severe flare-up.

Nutrition Facts

Servings: 2

Amount per serving

Calories	353
	% Daily Value*
Total Fat 30.4g	39%
Saturated Fat 6.7g	34%
Cholesterol 182mg	61%
Sodium 107mg	5%
Total Carbohydrate 9.6g	3%
Dietary Fiber 6.7g	24%
Total Sugars 1.4g	
Protein 13.5g	
Vitamin D 44mcg	220%
Calcium 26mg	2%
Iron 2mg	9%
Potassium 677mg	14%

BAKED APPLE

For those who have UC, cooked, and skin-removed fruits are great breakfast ingredients. You can use this recipe for cooking fruits like apple, peach, and pear.

- Prep Time: 5 minutes
- Cook Time: 40 minutes
- Total Time: 45 minutes
- Serving: 2

<u>Ingredients</u>

- 1 teaspoon cinnamon
- 1 teaspoon extra virgin olive oil
- 2 cups of water
- 2 tablespoons brown sugar

- 2 apples, cored

Instructions

1. In a medium/large pot, boil your apple with cinnamon, olive oil, water, and brown sugar over high heat for 40 minutes.
2. You can add more sugar for sweetness. However, it is not recommended for Ulcerative Colitis patients to add more sugar.
3. Remove the apple skin, and then, enjoy!

Cooking Tips:

- You can use the same instruction to make baked fruits such as pear or peach.

UC-related Tips:

- Do not use brown sugar during a flare-up or if it irritates your gut. Simply use stevia (one tablespoon) instead.

Nutrition Facts	
Servings: 2	
Amount per serving	
Calories	**173**
	% Daily Value*
Total Fat 2.7g	4%
Saturated Fat 0.3g	2%
Cholesterol 0mg	0%
Sodium 12mg	1%
Total Carbohydrate 40.8g	15%
Dietary Fiber 6g	21%
Total Sugars 32g	
Protein 0.7g	
Vitamin D 0mcg	0%
Calcium 27mg	2%
Iron 1mg	6%
Potassium 258mg	5%

PEAR OATMEAL BARS

A great source of fiber for those who have UC. This bar is gluten and lactose-free with a great taste of pear and ginger.

- Prep Time: 10 minutes
- Cook Time: 25 minutes
- Total Time: 35 minutes
- Serving: 4

Ingredients

- 4 organic pears
- ½ cup applesauce
- 1 teaspoon ground ginger
- ½ teaspoon salt
- ½ cup organic smooth almond butter
- 2 teaspoons pure vanilla extract
- 2 teaspoons ground cinnamon
- ¾ teaspoon baking powder
- ¾ cup oat flour (or gluten-free flour)
- ½ cup rolled oats (or a small package of ready oatmeal)

Instructions

1. Preheat oven to 375 °F.
2. Cook the pear or use a pear compote. Blend your pears to make a puree.
3. Mix your pear puree with applesauce, salt, almond butter, ginger, vanilla extract, cinnamon, baking powder, flour, and oats.
4. Pour your mix into a suitable oven pan.
5. Bake your oatmeal for 25 minutes until inside cooks well. Cut the baked oatmeal like bars.
6. Let it be cooled first and then serve!

<u>Cooking Tips:</u>

- It is recommended to use organic oats or ready oatmeal.
- To check if the inside cooks well, insert a toothpick inside. If it comes out without sticking to your bar, it shows that it cooked well.

<u>UC-related Tips:</u>

- Cook your pear or use pear compote if you cannot tolerate raw pear.
- If you have colon strictures due to UC, reduce your monthly oatmeal intakes.

Nutrition Facts

Servings: 4

Amount per serving

Calories	612
	% Daily Value*
Total Fat 34.2g	44%
Saturated Fat 3.4g	17%
Cholesterol 0mg	0%
Sodium 296mg	13%
Total Carbohydrate 70g	25%
Dietary Fiber 18.2g	65%
Total Sugars 27.9g	
Protein 14.6g	
Vitamin D 0mcg	0%
Calcium 249mg	19%
Iron 4mg	23%
Potassium 931mg	20%

AVOCADO & EGG BREAKFAST TOAST

A very simple, delicious breakfast dish, high in protein and healthy fat.

- Prep Time: 5 minutes
- Cook Time: 10 minutes
- Total Time: 15 minutes
- Serving: 2

Ingredients

- 4 slices of white toast or gluten-free bread
- ½ cup low fat cottage cheese or lactose-free Havarti cheese
- 1 avocado
- 2 large organic free-range eggs
- 4 egg whites
- 1 tablespoon lime juice
- Salt and pepper to taste

Instructions

1. Toast your white bread toasts the way you want.
2. Mix cheese, eggs, egg whites, salt, and pepper in a bowl and scramble it in a pan over medium heat for 7 minutes.
3. Coat your toasts with scrambled mix and mashed avocado. Then, squeeze lime. Enjoy!

Cooking Tips:

- You can use low-fat feta cheese instead of cottage cheese, as well.

UC-related Tips:

- Boil your eggs if you are experiencing a severe flare-up.
- Do not use black pepper if you are in a flare-up.

Nutrition Facts

Servings: 2

Amount per serving

Calories 411

	% Daily Value*
Total Fat 26.4g	34%
Saturated Fat 6.5g	32%
Cholesterol 191mg	64%
Sodium 467mg	20%
Total Carbohydrate 21.2g	8%
Dietary Fiber 7.2g	28%
Total Sugars 2.5g	
Protein 24.7g	
Vitamin D 18mcg	88%
Calcium 103mg	8%
Iron 2mg	12%
Potassium 751mg	16%

SMOOTHIE BOWL

A mix of skin-removed and chopped fruits can create a tremendous rich breakfast!

- Prep Time: 10 minutes
- Cook Time: 0 minutes
- Total Time: 10 minutes
- Serving: 2

Ingredients

- 1 banana, sliced
- 1 cup almond milk or lactose-free milk
- 1 cup pineapple chunks
- 1 cup diced mango

Instructions

1. Blend all mentioned ingredients in a blender. Serve and Enjoy!

Cooking Tips:

- You can use the same instruction to make fruit bowls with other fruits you can tolerate.

- You can add 1 cup of papaya to your bowl as well.

UC-related Tips:

- Use ¼ mango if you are experiencing a severe flare-up or, instead, use 1 cup of papaya.

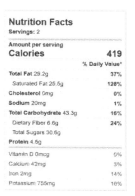

Nutrition Facts	
Servings: 2	
Amount per serving	
Calories	**419**
	% Daily Value*
Total Fat 29.2g	37%
Saturated Fat 25.5g	128%
Cholesterol 0mg	0%
Sodium 20mg	1%
Total Carbohydrate 43.3g	16%
Dietary Fiber 6.6g	24%
Total Sugars 30.6g	
Protein 4.5g	
Vitamin D 0mcg	0%
Calcium 42mg	3%
Iron 2mg	14%
Potassium 755mg	16%

ZUCCHINI BREAD OATMEAL

Enjoy the taste of grated zucchini and oatmeal and have a healthy UC adapted breakfast!

- Prep Time: 5 minutes
- Cook Time: 7 minutes
- Total Time: 12 minutes
- Serving: 2

Ingredients

- ⅓ cup organic rolled oats or ready oatmeal
- 1 cup unsweetened almond or lactose-free milk
- ½ teaspoon cinnamon powder
- ½ cup zucchini
- 1 teaspoon vanilla extract
- Maple syrup (optional)

Instructions

1. Mix your milk with cinnamon and oat in a medium pot and boil the mixture over medium heat for 4 minutes.
2. Grate zucchini, add it to the mix, and stir well for three minutes.
3. In a small bowl, mix vanilla extract and maple syrup.
4. When oatmeal cooked, remove from heat and pour the syrup on it.
5. Let it be cooled and then serve!

Cooking Tips:

- You can use maple or agave syrup in this recipe if you can tolerate it.

UC-related Tips:

- If you have colon strictures due to UC, reduce your monthly oatmeal intakes. Avoid any types of seeds.

Nutrition Facts	
Servings: 2	
Amount per serving	
Calories	**82**
	% Daily Value*
Total Fat 2.7g	3%
Saturated Fat 0.3g	2%
Cholesterol 0mg	0%
Sodium 94mg	4%
Total Carbohydrate 11.5g	4%
Dietary Fiber 2.2g	8%
Total Sugars 0.9g	
Protein 2.6g	
Vitamin D 1mcg	3%
Calcium 182mg	12%
Iron 1mg	8%
Potassium 222mg	5%

BREAKFAST FRUIT SALAD

A mix of a variety of fruits (skin-removed and chopped) can create an excellent breakfast salad for Ulcerative Colitis patients!

- Prep Time: 5 minutes
- Cook Time: 25 minutes
- Total Time: 30 minutes
- Serving: 6

Ingredients

- 1 can pineapple chunks
- 2 large firm bananas, cubed
- 1 medium mango, skin removed and cubed
- 1 medium green apple, skin removed and cubed
- 1 medium papaya, skin-removed and cubed
- 1 tablespoon lemon juice
- ½ cup sugar or 1 tablespoon stevia (optional)
- ⅓ cup orange juice (optional)

Instructions

1. Mix all fruits in a bowl.
2. Boil your orange juice, lemon juice, and sugar in a small pot (over high heat). Stir well.
3. Let the juice be cooled. Then, add your cooled juice to the fruit bowl. Enjoy!

Cooking Tips:

- You can use orange juice in this recipe if you can tolerate it.

UC-related Tips:

- If you are experiencing a severe flare-up, cook your fruits first.

Nutrition Facts

Servings: 6

Amount per serving	
Calories	**108**

	% Daily Value*
Total Fat 0.4g	1%
Saturated Fat 0.1g	1%
Cholesterol 0mg	0%
Sodium 6mg	0%
Total Carbohydrate 27.7g	10%
Dietary Fiber 3.5g	13%
Total Sugars 18.8g	
Protein 1g	
Vitamin D 0mcg	0%
Calcium 17mg	1%
Iron 1mg	3%
Potassium 331mg	7%

BANANA SPLIT OATMEAL

A great combination of oatmeal and banana can make a great breakfast full of fiber and potassium.

- Prep Time: 10 minutes
- Cook Time: 0 minutes
- Total Time: 10 minutes
- Serving: 2

Ingredients

- ½ cup water, almond milk or lactose-free milk
- 1 cup old-fashioned rolled oats or a small ready oatmeal package
- ½ banana, cubed
- Salt to taste

Instructions

1. Boil your milk or water in a pot over high heat.
2. Add oat and salt to it. Stir for two more minutes.

3. Serve your oatmeal with cubed bananas. Enjoy!

Cooking Tips:

- You can use honey, maple or agave syrup in this recipe if you can tolerate.

UC-related Tips:

- If you have colon strictures due to UC, reduce your monthly oatmeal intakes.

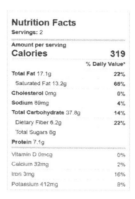

Nutrition Facts

Servings: 2

Amount per serving

Calories	319
	% Daily Value*
Total Fat 17.1g	22%
Saturated Fat 13.2g	68%
Cholesterol 0mg	0%
Sodium 89mg	4%
Total Carbohydrate 37.8g	14%
Dietary Fiber 6.2g	22%
Total Sugars 8g	
Protein 7.1g	
Vitamin D 0mcg	0%
Calcium 32mg	2%
Iron 3mg	16%
Potassium 412mg	9%

EGG TACOS WITH AVOCADO

Enjoy a breakfast sandwich with egg and avocado, which is full of healthy fats and functional proteins.

- Prep Time: 5 minutes
- Cook Time: 10 minutes
- Total Time: 15 minutes
- Serving: 2

Ingredients

- 4 small tortillas
- 2 organic, free-range eggs

- 1 avocado
- Salt to taste

Instructions

1. Warm or toast tortillas.
2. Scramble or boil your eggs using salt.
3. Mash your avocado
4. Fill your tortillas with avocado and eggs. Enjoy!

Cooking Tips:

- You can use white bread or gluten-free bread (if you can tolerate them) instead of tortillas.

UC-related Tips:

- If you have colon strictures or flare-up due to UC, use very soft bread with white flour-like a white pita. If you are sensitive to gluten, use soft gluten-free white rice bread.

Nutrition Facts

Servings: 2

Amount per serving

Calories	373
	% Daily Value*
Total Fat 25.3g	32%
Saturated Fat 5.7g	29%
Cholesterol 164mg	55%
Sodium 167mg	7%
Total Carbohydrate 30.4g	11%
Dietary Fiber 9.8g	35%
Total Sugars 1.3g	
Protein 10.2g	
Vitamin D 15mcg	77%
Calcium 74mg	6%
Iron 2mg	11%
Potassium 636mg	14%

CRISPY HASH BROWN WITH EGG

Start your day with hash brown and egg! A great combination, as always!

- Prep Time: 20 minutes
- Cook Time: 15 minutes
- Total Time: 35 minutes
- Serving: 2

Ingredients

- 2 large yellow potatoes, shredded
- ¼ cup all-purpose flour or gluten-free flour
- 2 tablespoons extra virgin olive oil
- 2 organic range-free eggs
- Salt and pepper to taste

Instructions

1. Shred potatoes and rinse them until the water cleared. Dry potatoes.
2. Mix your potatoes with flour, eggs, salt, and pepper.
3. Flatten your mix in a large skillet and let it cook over medium heat until golden brown. Flip and cook the other side.
4. Remove from the skillet and drain with a paper towel. Enjoy!

Cooking Tips:

- To flip it quickly, you can cut in half or quarter.

UC-related Tips:

- Do not use pepper if you are experiencing a severe flare-up. Try to boil and mash your potatoes as well.

Nutrition Facts

Servings: 2

Amount per serving

Calories 385

	% Daily Value*
Total Fat 18.7g	24%
Saturated Fat 3.4g	17%
Cholesterol 164mg	55%
Sodium 70mg	3%
Total Carbohydrate 45.8g	17%
Dietary Fiber 2.8g	10%
Total Sugars 3g	
Protein 10.2g	
Vitamin D 15mcg	77%
Calcium 34mg	3%
Iron 2mg	12%
Potassium 686mg	15%

GRILLED ALMOND BUTTER HONEY BANANA SANDWICH

An excellent easy to make a sandwich for your breakfast.

- Prep Time: 5 minutes
- Cook Time: 0 minutes
- Total Time: 5 minutes
- Serving: 2

Ingredients

- 1 tablespoon extra virgin olive oil
- Few grams of almond butter
- 1 banana
- 4 slices of white bread or gluten-free bread
- Honey or maple syrup to taste

Instructions

- Toast your bread slices, as you desired.
- Mash banana, coat your bread with banana, almond butter, and honey (maple syrup). Enjoy!

Cooking Tips:

- You can use honey, maple or agave syrup in this recipe if you can tolerate.

UC-related Tips:

- If you have colon stricture(s) due to UC, make sure you are using smoothened types of almond butter.

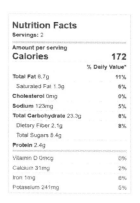

Nutrition Facts	
Servings: 2	
Amount per serving	
Calories	**172**
	% Daily Value*
Total Fat 8.7g	11%
Saturated Fat 1.5g	6%
Cholesterol 0mg	0%
Sodium 123mg	5%
Total Carbohydrate 23.3g	8%
Dietary Fiber 2.1g	8%
Total Sugars 9.4g	
Protein 2.4g	
Vitamin D 0mcg	0%
Calcium 31mg	2%
Iron 1mg	6%
Potassium 241mg	5%

AVOCADO-CHEESE BAGEL

If you are in love with a bagel, you will enjoy making an avocado-cheese bagel recipe.

- Prep Time: 5 minutes
- Cook Time: 0 minutes
- Total Time: 5 minutes
- Serving: 1

Ingredients

- 1 white bagel or gluten-free bread, toasted
- 2 tablespoons low-fat feta cheese or lactose-free Swiss cheese
- ½ avocado, mashed
- Salt to taste

Instructions

- Open the bagel and coat a half with cheese, avocado (mashed), and salt.
- Cover with the other half. Enjoy!

Cooking Tips:

- Use bagels with white flour.
- You may want to add fresh lemon juice to your avocado for another great taste and avoid turning avocado to brown.

UC-related Tips:

- If you have colon strictures due to UC, make sure you are using seedless bagels.

Nutrition Facts

Servings: 1

Amount per serving	
Calories	**525**
	% Daily Value*
Total Fat 21.3g	27%
Saturated Fat 4.4g	22%
Cholesterol 3mg	1%
Sodium 896mg	39%
Total Carbohydrate 66.2g	24%
Dietary Fiber 9.3g	33%
Total Sugars 6.3g	
Protein 19.9g	
Vitamin D 0mcg	0%
Calcium 210mg	16%
Iron 5mg	28%
Potassium 572mg	12%

PINEAPPLE-GINGER OATMEAL

Another great recipe for oatmeal with amazing mix flavors of ginger and pineapple.

- Prep Time: 5 minutes
- Cook Time: 20 minutes
- Total Time: 25 minutes

- Serving: 4

Ingredients

- 2 cups old-fashioned rolled oats
- 2 cups pineapple chunks
- 1 small piece of ginger or one teaspoon ginger powder
- ½ teaspoon salt
- 2 cups unsweetened almond or lactose-free milk
- ½ cups honey or maple syrup
- 2 large organic free-range eggs
- 2 teaspoon vanilla extract

Instructions

- Preheat oven to 375 °F.
- In a medium bowl, mix and whisk oats with ginger, salt, pineapple, and milk.
- Use a suitable baking pan or sheet. Spread your mix to it and bake for 20 minutes until golden brown.

Cooking Tips:

- You can prepare this breakfast in a large skillet over medium heat until brown.
- Use agave syrup or one teaspoon of stevia if you cannot tolerate maple syrup or honey.

UC-related Tips:

- If you have colon strictures due to UC, make sure you are using less oatmeal monthly.

Nutrition Facts

Servings: 4

Amount per serving

Calories 308

	% Daily Value*
Total Fat 5.6g	7%
Saturated Fat 1.2g	6%
Cholesterol 93mg	31%
Sodium 419mg	18%
Total Carbohydrate 61g	22%
Dietary Fiber 3.8g	14%
Total Sugars 43.9g	
Protein 6.8g	
Vitamin D 9mcg	47%
Calcium 177mg	14%
Iron 2mg	12%
Potassium 250mg	5%

APPLE CINNAMON OATMEAL

Enjoy tasting a traditional apple cinnamon oatmeal that can be prepared in less than 15 minutes.

- Prep Time: 5 minutes
- Cook Time: 15 minutes
- Total Time: 20 minutes
- Serving: 2

Ingredients

- 1 tablespoon extra virgin olive oil
- 1 cup gluten-free ground oats or ready oatmeal
- 2 cups unsweetened almond or lactose-free milk
- ½ teaspoon cinnamon
- 1 large apple, sliced and skin-removed
- 1 tablespoon maple syrup, or agave syrup
- ¼ cup pomegranate juice (optional)

Instructions

- Preheat oven to 375 °F.

- In a medium bowl, mix and whisk oats with cinnamon, oil, apple, pomegranate juice (optional), maple syrup, and milk.
- Use a suitable baking pan or sheet. Spread your mix to it and bake for 15 minutes until golden brown.

Cooking Tips:

- You can prepare this breakfast in a large skillet over medium heat for 10-15 minutes until brown.
- Use agave syrup or 1 teaspoon of stevia if you cannot tolerate maple syrup or honey.

UC-related Tips:

- If you have colon strictures due to UC, make sure you are using less oatmeal monthly.
- Use pomegranate juice only if you can tolerate it.
- If you are experiencing a flare-up, cook your apple first.

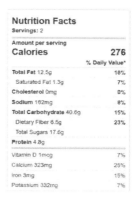

Nutrition Facts	
Servings: 2	
Amount per serving	
Calories	**276**
	% Daily Value*
Total Fat 12.5g	16%
Saturated Fat 1.3g	7%
Cholesterol 0mg	0%
Sodium 182mg	8%
Total Carbohydrate 40.6g	15%
Dietary Fiber 6.5g	23%
Total Sugars 17.6g	
Protein 4.8g	
Vitamin D 1mcg	7%
Calcium 323mg	25%
Iron 3mg	15%
Potassium 332mg	7%

APPETIZERS

TURKEY POTPIE SOUP

Great soup with perfect ingredients for Ulcerative Colitis patients.

- Prep Time: 10 minutes
- Cook Time: 35 minutes
- Total Time: 45 minutes
- Serving: 4

Ingredients

- ¼ cup white gluten-free flour or refined all-purpose flour
- 16 oz turkey breast, cubed
- 2 cups turkey/chicken stock, divided
- 4 cups fat-free milk or lactose-free cow milk
- 1 teaspoon turmeric powder
- 2 celery stalks, chopped in small pieces
- 1 large carrot, cubed 1 inch (~2.54 cm)
- 2 medium potatoes, peeled and cubed 1 inch (~2.54 cm)
- Salt and pepper, to taste

Instructions

1. Mix 1 cup of turkey/chicken broth with flour and whisk well. Set aside.
2. Pour another cup of broth into a large pot. Add turkey, celery, potatoes and turmeric powder inside and boil until vegetables and turkey get soft.
3. Warm milk and add to the mix. Then, add carrots and cook for another 5 minutes. Add salt and pepper to taste.

Cooking Tips:

- You may want to add one cup of mushroom if you can tolerate it.
- You can remove flour from the recipe if you do not have one or do not want a soup with a thick texture.
- You can make this soup with chicken breasts as well.

UC-related Tips:

- If you cannot tolerate ordinary mushrooms, you may try Shiitake mushroom.
- Do not use pepper if you are experiencing a severe flare-up.

Nutrition Facts

Servings: 4

Amount per serving

Calories 326

	% Daily Value*
Total Fat 2.4g	3%
Saturated Fat 0.5g	3%
Cholesterol 54mg	18%
Sodium 1696mg	74%
Total Carbohydrate 42.3g	15%
Dietary Fiber 4.2g	15%
Total Sugars 18.6g	
Protein 30.6g	
Vitamin D 1mcg	6%
Calcium 341mg	26%
Iron 3mg	16%
Potassium 1266mg	27%

POTATO-GINGER MISO SOUP

A fabulous Miso soup with GI healing ingredients. A great source of required vitamins and minerals for Ulcerative Colitis patients:

- Prep Time: 10 minutes
- Cook Time: 30 minutes
- Total Time: 40 minutes
- Serving: 3-4

Ingredients

- 1 fresh ginger or ½ tablespoon fresh grated ginger
- 2 cups sodium-free/low sodium vegetable broth
- 2 tablespoons miso
- 2 medium potatoes, peeled and cubed 1 inch (~2.54 cm)
- ½ cup unsweetened almond milk
- ½ teaspoon salt
- ½ teaspoon garlic powder (optional)

Instructions

1. Boil potatoes in a medium pot until softened.
2. Drain and mash your potatoes.
3. In a medium/large pot, mix broth, ginger, salt, and garlic powder (optional) and boil over medium heat.
4. Add mashed potatoes to the mix and blend until smoothened.
5. Add warm miso and almond milk. Blend again until smoothened. Then, heat the soup for 5 more minutes over medium heat. Enjoy!

Cooking Tips:

- You can add 1 cup of chicken breast to the recipe if you want to have chicken miso.

UC-related Tips:

- Do not use garlic powder if you cannot tolerate it, or you are experiencing a severe flare-up.

Nutrition Facts

Servings: 3

Amount per serving

Calories   **242**

	% Daily Value*
Total Fat 11.3g	15%
Saturated Fat 8.9g	45%
Cholesterol 0mg	0%
Sodium 961mg	41%
Total Carbohydrate 28.8g	10%
Dietary Fiber 5g	18%
Total Sugars 4.2g	
Protein 8g	
Vitamin D 0mcg	0%
Calcium 33mg	3%
Iron 2mg	12%
Potassium 857mg	18%

PARSNIP/CARROT POTATO SOUP

The parsnip is a root vegetable from the carrot family. Do not use parsnip if you are in a flare-up. Instead, use carrot in the recipe.

- Prep Time: 10 minutes
- Cook Time: 30 minutes
- Total Time: 40 minutes
- Serving: 4

Ingredients

- 1 celery stalk, chopped
- 4 parsnips or carrots, cubed 1 inch (~2.54 cm)
- 3 cups chicken broth
- 1 tablespoon extra virgin olive oil
- 2 potatoes, skin removed and cubed 1 inch (~2.54 cm)
- 1 teaspoon salt
- 2 tablespoons low-fat feta cheese or lactose-free Havarti cheese (optional)
- 1 teaspoon pepper (optional)

Instructions

6. Choose a large pan and cook celery and parsnip (carrot) using extra virgin olive oil over medium heat and occasionally mix until semi-soft texture.
7. Warm up the broth and pour it into the pan. Add potato, salt, and pepper (optional) and cook for 20 minutes.
8. Enjoy the soup as it is or blend it for having a puree.
9. Sprinkle low-fat feta cheese or lactose-free Havarti cheese on top if you desire.

Cooking Tips:

- You can mix all ingredients at the same time and let it boil for 25-30 minutes.

UC-related Tips:

- Do not use parsnip if you cannot tolerate it, or you are experiencing a severe flare-up. Instead, use carrots.
- Do not use pepper if you are experiencing a severe flare-up.

Nutrition Facts
Servings: 4

Amount per serving
Calories 184

	% Daily Value*
Total Fat 4.9g	8%
Saturated Fat 0.9g	4%
Cholesterol 0mg	0%
Sodium 583mg	26%
Total Carbohydrate 29.7g	11%
Dietary Fiber 8g	21%
Total Sugars 5.1g	
Protein 6.3g	
Vitamin D 0mcg	0%
Calcium 46mg	3%
Iron 1mg	7%
Potassium 864mg	18%

PUMPKIN SOUP

Great semi-classical pumpkin soup can be one of your choices to make every week.

- Prep Time: 15 minutes
- Cook Time: 15 minutes
- Total Time: 30 minutes
- Serving: 4-6

Ingredients

- 2 lbs (~1 kg) pumpkin, skin-removed, seeds-removed, chopped
- 1 large carrot, skin-removed, diced
- 2 large potatoes, skin removed, diced
- 4 cups sodium-free/low sodium chicken broth
- ½ cup milk or lactose-free cow milk
- Salt and pepper, to taste
- 2 chicken bouillon cubes (optional)
- 1 tablespoon garlic powder (optional)

Instructions

1. Mix and boil all ingredients in a large pot over medium heat.
2. Remove from heat. Blend the soup until smooth.
3. Add salt, and pepper to taste

Cooking Tips:

- If you can tolerate and if you can find a very light cream/sour cream, you can use it instead of milk.
- If you are in remission, you can cook vegetables first in a large skillet by 1 tablespoon extra virgin olive oil over medium heat until semi-soft texture. Then, boil and blend.

<u>UC-related Tips:</u>

- Do not use pepper if you are experiencing a severe flare-up.

Nutrition Facts
Servings: 6

Amount per serving

Calories   **174**

	% Daily Value*
Total Fat 1.5g	2%
Saturated Fat 0.5g	3%
Cholesterol 0mg	0%
Sodium 543mg	24%
Total Carbohydrate 34.3g	12%
Dietary Fiber 7.6g	27%
Total Sugars 8.5g	
Protein 7.8g	
Vitamin D 0mcg	1%
Calcium 86mg	7%
Iron 3mg	17%
Potassium 988mg	21%

STRACCIATELLA SOUP

This delicious Italian soup is entirely in line with Ulcerative Colitis patient tolerance levels full of healthy ingredients. It can significantly supply your protein.

- Prep Time: 10 minutes
- Cook Time: 15 minutes
- Total Time: 25 minutes
- Serving: 4

<u>Ingredients</u>

- 6 cups low sodium/sodium-free chicken broth
- 2 tablespoons semolina flour or all-purpose gluten-free flour
- 3 large organic free-range eggs
- Salt and pepper, to taste
- 1 tablespoon hard pecorino cheese, grated

- 1 tablespoon hard Parmigiano-Reggiano cheese, grated
- 1 tablespoon fresh parsley (optional)

Instructions

1. In a large pot and over high heat, bring chicken stock to simmer. Add salt and pepper.
2. In a large bowl, whisk eggs, semolina or all-purpose gluten-free flour, Parmigiano-Reggiano, and pecorino cheese altogether.
3. Slowly pour the egg mixture into your pot and simmer well. Let the soup simmer.
4. Serve and garnish it with parsley if you want. Enjoy!

Cooking Tips:

- Most aged cheddar-type cheese is lactose-free. As such, lactose-intolerant patients can tolerate pecorino and Parmigiano-Reggiano. However, they should be used in moderation during a flare-up.

UC-related Tips:

- Use pecorino and Parmigiano-Reggiano in moderation if you are in a flare-up or simply remove them from the recipe.
- Do not use pepper if you are experiencing a severe flare-up.

Nutrition Facts

Servings: 4

Amount per serving

Calories   **164**

	% Daily Value*
Total Fat 8.3g	11%
Saturated Fat 3.5g	18%
Cholesterol 147mg	49%
Sodium 1277mg	56%
Total Carbohydrate 5.5g	2%
Dietary Fiber 0.2g	1%
Total Sugars 1.3g	
Protein 15.4g	
Vitamin D 13mcg	66%
Calcium 120mg	9%
Iron 2mg	9%
Potassium 376mg	8%

HAM AND POTATO SOUP

A delicious soup for Ulcerative Colitis patients who love ham.

- Prep Time: 10 minutes
- Cook Time: 20 minutes
- Total Time: 30 minutes
- Serving: 4

Ingredients

- 2 large potatoes, peeled and cubed 1 inch (~2.54 cm)
- 1 cup cooked ham, diced and cubed 1 inch (~2.54 cm)
- 3 cups sodium-free/low sodium chicken broth
- 1 tablespoon extra virgin olive oil
- ¼ cup white all-purpose flour or gluten-free flour
- ½ cup celery stalk, diced
- 2 cups milk, or lactose-free cow milk
- Salt and pepper to taste

Instructions

1. Boil potatoes, celery, ham, and chicken broth in a large pot over medium heat for 15 minutes.
2. In a large pan, pour high-quality extra virgin olive oil and whisk flour over medium heat. Stir consistently until golden brown. Warm milk and add slowly to the flour. Stir continuously for five minutes.
3. Pour the mix into the pot and stir. Add salt and pepper to taste. Enjoy!

Cooking Tips:

- For having a classic taste, you can use honey ham.

UC-related Tips:

- If you are in a severe flare-up, avoid using ham/honey ham. Instead, use fat-removed pork tenderloin or chicken breasts.
- Do not use pepper if you are experiencing a severe flare-up.

Nutrition Facts

Servings: 4

Amount per serving

Calories	316
	% Daily Value*
Total Fat 9.2g	12%
Saturated Fat 3.1g	15%
Cholesterol 29mg	10%
Sodium 935mg	41%
Total Carbohydrate 43.3g	16%
Dietary Fiber 5.3g	19%
Total Sugars 8.2g	
Protein 16.1g	
Vitamin D 1mcg	3%
Calcium 190mg	15%
Iron 2mg	12%
Potassium 1112mg	24%

BUTTERNUT SQUASH SOUP

A perfect soup for people with UC to be included in their weekly diet.

- Prep Time: 10 minutes
- Cook Time: 55 minutes
- Total Time: 65 minutes
- Serving: 6

Ingredients

- 3 lbs (~1.5 kg) butternut squash, halved & skin-removed
- 2 carrots, peeled and cubed
- 3-4 cups low sodium chicken or vegetable stock/broth
- 2 chicken or beef bouillon cubes
- ¼ cup olive oil (for roasting option)
- 2 teaspoons salt, to taste
- 1 teaspoon garlic powder (optional)
- 1 teaspoon ground black pepper, to taste (optional)

Instructions

1. Boil all ingredients in a large pot over medium heat for 40 minutes until softened. Remove from the pot. Allow to cool down for 5-10 minutes.
2. Pour all ingredients into a blender. Then, blend until smooth. Serve hot and enjoy!

Cooking Tips:

- For having a classic taste, you can use low-fat cream/sour cream on top if you can tolerate it.
- Be careful with the steam that may come out of the blended soup.

UC-related Tips:

- Do not use pepper or garlic powder if you are experiencing a severe flare-up.

Nutrition Facts

Servings: 6

Amount per serving	
Calories	**193**
	% Daily Value*
Total Fat 8.7g	11%
Saturated Fat 1.3g	7%
Cholesterol 0mg	0%
Sodium 1037mg	45%
Total Carbohydrate 29.3g	11%
Dietary Fiber 5g	18%
Total Sugars 6.2g	
Protein 3.6g	
Vitamin D 0mcg	0%
Calcium 117mg	9%
Iron 2mg	10%
Potassium 669mg	18%

CHICKEN NOODLE SOUP

The chicken noodle soup is one of the famed soups all around the world. Enjoy making it in less than 45 minutes!

- Prep Time: 5 minutes
- Cook Time: 40 minutes
- Total Time: 45 minutes
- Serving: 6

Ingredients

- 1 cup vermicelli or egg noodles or rice noodles (gluten-free option)
- 8 skin-removed chicken legs
- 1-2 chicken bouillon cube(s), crushed
- 2 cups of water
- 1 tablespoon extra virgin olive oil
- 2 teaspoons salt, to taste
- 2 large carrots, cubed & skin-removed
- 1 celery stalk, chopped

- 6 cups low sodium chicken stock/broth
- 1 teaspoon garlic powder (optional)
- 1 teaspoon ground black pepper, to taste (optional)
- ¼ cup fresh parsley, chopped (optional)

Instructions

1. In a large skillet, heat high-quality olive oil over medium heat and cook celery and carrots for 5 minutes.
2. Pour chicken broth into the skillet, add and cook chicken legs.
3. Add crushed bouillons and water to cover all ingredients.
4. When chicken cooked, use a plate to shred it and remove the bone.
5. Bring shredded chickens back to the soup and add noodles. Add salt, pepper, and garlic powder (optional). Cover it for 7 minutes. Then, open the lid and stir well.
6. Serve in a bowl and garnish with chopped fresh parsley (optional)

Cooking Tips:

- You can use skin-removed chicken thighs or breasts instead of chicken legs, as well.
- You can use gluten-free noodles if you are gluten-intolerant.

UC-related Tips:

- Do not use pepper or garlic powder or parsley if you are experiencing a severe flare-up.

Nutrition Facts

Servings: 6

Amount per serving

Calories   **420**

	% Daily Value*
Total Fat 13.9g	18%
Saturated Fat 3.3g	17%
Cholesterol 120mg	40%
Sodium 1175mg	51%
Total Carbohydrate 26.3g	10%
Dietary Fiber 1.6g	6%
Total Sugars 3.2g	
Protein 41.9g	
Vitamin D 0mcg	0%
Calcium 27mg	2%
Iron 3mg	19%
Potassium 346mg	7%

CREAMY CHICKEN SOUP

A very delicious savory soup specially modified for Ulcerative Colitis patients.

- Prep Time: 5 minutes
- Cook Time: 30 minutes
- Total Time: 35 minutes
- Serving: 4-6

Ingredients

- 1.5 lbs boneless, skin-removed chicken breast
- 1 cup carrots, skin-removed and cubed 1 inch (~2.54 cm)
- 1 medium potato, skin-removed and cubed 1 inch (~2.54 cm)
- 2 tablespoons extra virgin olive oil
- 1 cup low-fat milk or lactose-free cow milk
- 3 cups low-sodium chicken broth
- 1 teaspoon turmeric powder
- Salt and pepper, to taste
- ½ teaspoon dried thyme
- 1-2 tablespoon(s) lemon juice

- 1 teaspoon garlic powder (optional)
- 1 cup mushrooms (optional)
- 1 cup cream/sour cream (optional)

Instructions

1. Heat extra virgin olive oil in a large pot and cook chicken over medium heat with turmeric, salt, and pepper until golden brown both sides. Remove chickens.
2. Add carrots, potato, thyme, garlic powder (optional), and mushroom (optional) to the pot. Stir well until half-cooked. Add chicken broth. Then, let it cook for 15-20 minutes.
3. Add warm milk and 1-2 tablespoon(s) lemon juice. Let it simmer for five more minutes. Serve warm and enjoy!

Cooking Tips:

- You can use ½ cup shiitake mushroom if regular mushrooms irritate your gut, or remove mushroom from the recipe.
- You can add sour cream on top of the soup if you can tolerate it during remissions.

UC-related Tips:

- Do not use pepper or garlic powder if you are experiencing a severe flare-up.
- If you are in extreme flare-up condition, boil chicken as well.

Nutrition Facts

Servings: 6

Amount per serving

Calories	224

% Daily Value*

Total Fat 6.7g	9%
Saturated Fat 1g	5%
Cholesterol 66mg	23%
Sodium 145mg	6%
Total Carbohydrate 10.9g	4%
Dietary Fiber 1.4g	5%
Total Sugars 3.4g	
Protein 29.8g	
Vitamin D 21mcg	106%
Calcium 61mg	5%
Iron 2mg	8%
Potassium 285mg	6%

SEAFOOD CHOWDER SOUP

A must-try recipe if you are in love with seafood!

- Prep Time: 10 minutes
- Cook Time: 25 minutes
- Total Time: 35 minutes
- Serving: 4-6

Ingredients

- 3 potatoes, peeled and cubed 1 inch (~2.54 cm)
- 2 cups of low-sodium vegetable broth or chicken broth
- ¾ cup of milk, or lactose-free cow milk
- 4 oz salmon filet, peeled and cubed
- 4 oz codfish filet, peeled and cubed
- 8 raw shrimps, peeled
- 2 tablespoons fresh lemon juice
- 1 bay leaf
- ½ teaspoon grated ginger
- Salt and pepper to taste
- 2 tablespoons of apple cider vinegar (optional)

Instructions

1. In a large pot, warm chicken broth and add potatoes, bay leaf, apple cider vinegar (optional), salmon, and cod.
2. Let the soup cook for 15 minutes over medium heat. Stir occasionally. Cover but leave a corner open for the steam to escape.
3. Add warm milk, shrimp, lemon juice, ginger, sale, and pepper to the soup. Stir for 5-10 minutes. Enjoy!

Cooking Tips:

- You can add ⅓ cup of crab into the soup if you like.
- You can add sour cream on top of the soup if you can tolerate it.

UC-related Tips:

- Do not use pepper if you are experiencing a severe flare-up.

Nutrition Facts

Servings: 6

Amount per serving

Calories	268
	% Daily Value*
Total Fat 7.1g	9%
Saturated Fat 1.6g	8%
Cholesterol 134mg	45%
Sodium 265mg	12%
Total Carbohydrate 20.5g	7%
Dietary Fiber 3g	11%
Total Sugars 3.7g	
Protein 31.4g	
Vitamin D 0mcg	1%
Calcium 112mg	9%
Iron 2mg	10%
Potassium 772mg	16%

BARLEY/OATMEAL SOUP

A delicious Mediterranean soup with healthy, rich ingredients for Ulcerative Colitis patients!

- Prep Time: 10 minutes
- Soak Time: 120 minutes
- Cook Time: 40 minutes
- Total Time: 50 (or 170) minutes
- Serving: 6

Ingredients

- 1 cup barley or oatmeal
- 1 tablespoon all-purpose white flour or gluten-free flour
- 1.5 cup low-fat milk or lactose-free cow milk
- 1 cup carrot, peeled and cubed 1 inch (~2.54 cm)
- 7 cups low-sodium chicken broth
- 1 tablespoon extra virgin olive oil
- 1 tablespoon fresh lemon, squeezed
- Salt & pepper, to taste
- 1 tablespoon parsley, chopped (optional)

Instructions

1. First, let the barley soak for 2 hours. You can use oatmeal if you do not want to wait for 2 hours.
2. In a large pot, cook barley (or oatmeal) and carrots with chicken broth over medium heat for 30 minutes. Add salt and pepper. Stir occasionally.
3. In a medium pan, make a béchamel sauce: heat extra virgin olive oil. Add flour to the oil and stir until golden brown. Slowly add warm milk to the pan and stir perfectly until thickened. If the sauce is very thick, add more milk.

4. Add béchamel sauce to the pot and add lemon juice. Stir well over low heat for 5-10 more minutes.
5. Garnish the top with chopped parsley. Enjoy!

Cooking Tips:

- You may want to add ½ cup skin-removed chicken breast to your soup to make a chicken-barley soup.
- An orange-color barley soup can be made by one tablespoon tomato paste and 1 cup of water instead of 1.5 cups of milk.

UC-related Tips:

- Do not use pepper and parsley if you are experiencing a severe flare-up.
- If you cannot tolerate tomato, do not use the orange version of this soup explained in the cooking tips section.

Nutrition Facts

Servings: 6

Amount per serving

Calories	185
	% Daily Value*
Total Fat 3.7g	5%
Saturated Fat 0.8g	4%
Cholesterol 3mg	1%
Sodium 125mg	5%
Total Carbohydrate 29.6g	11%
Dietary Fiber 5.9g	21%
Total Sugars 4.4g	
Protein 8.5g	
Vitamin D 32mcg	159%
Calcium 89mg	7%
Iron 2mg	9%
Potassium 293mg	6%

LENTIL SOUP

A great healthy and easy to cook middle-eastern soup for Ulcerative Colitis patients during the remission period.

- Prep Time: 5 minutes
- Cook Time: 45 minutes
- Total Time: 50 minutes
- Serving: 4

Ingredients

- ¾ cup green lentils, washed
- 3 cups low-sodium chicken broth or water
- 1 tablespoon extra virgin olive oil
- ½ tablespoon salt, to taste
- ½ tablespoon turmeric powder
- 1 teaspoon cinnamon powder
- ½ teaspoon pepper (optional)
- 1 teaspoon garlic powder (optional)
- 1 teaspoon Angelica powder (optional)

Instructions

1. Choose a large pot and put all ingredients, except Angelica and cinnamon powder into it. Add water or chicken broth and let it boil over high heat.
2. Cover but stir occasionally. Let the lentils cook for 40 minutes over low/medium heat.
3. Add angelical and cinnamon powders. Enjoy!

Cooking Tips:

- You may want to add ½ cup skin-removed chicken breast to your recipe to make a chicken-lentil soup.
- You can blend the soup to have a smooth texture.

UC-related Tips:

- Do not use pepper and garlic powder if you are experiencing a severe flare-up.

- Use lentil in moderation and cook this recipe only during remissions. It can cause bloating in some patients. Avoid using this soup when you are experiencing a flare-up. Alternatively, you can remove lentils and consume the clear broth.

Nutrition Facts

Servings: 4

Amount per serving

Calories	171
	% Daily Value*
Total Fat 4g	5%
Saturated Fat 0.6g	3%
Cholesterol 0mg	0%
Sodium 927mg	40%
Total Carbohydrate 22.9g	8%
Dietary Fiber 11.2g	40%
Total Sugars 0.8g	
Protein 10.9g	
Vitamin D 0mcg	0%
Calcium 22mg	2%
Iron 3mg	19%
Potassium 365mg	8%

HOMEMADE VEGETABLE BROTH

It is an excellent idea for people living with UC to make their homemade vegetable broth instead of purchasing it from the stores. Many vegetable products are high in sodium and are mixed vegetables that cannot be well-tolerated by Ulcerative Colitis patients.

- Prep Time: 10 minutes
- Cook Time: 45 minutes
- Total Time: 55 minutes
- Serving: 4-6

<u>Ingredients</u>

- 4 cups celery, chopped
- 4 cups carrot, skin-removed and cubed
- 4 cups of water
- 2 tablespoons fresh lemon juice

- 2 tablespoons extra virgin olive oil
- ½ tablespoon turmeric powder
- 1 bay leaf
- ½ tablespoon salt, to taste
- 1 tablespoon fresh parsley, chopped (optional)
- ½ teaspoon pepper (optional)
- 1 teaspoon garlic powder (optional)

Instructions

1. Choose a large pan and cook vegetables with extra virgin olive oil, turmeric powder, salt, and pepper over medium heat until golden brown.
2. Put ingredients in the pan into a large pot, add water, lemon juice, bay leaf, garlic powder (optional), and chopped fresh parsley (optional). Thoroughly boil over low heat until all ingredients get soft.
3. Clear the broth by a colander. Serve immediately or pour and store in a suitable bottle for further use.

Cooking Tips:

- You can blend all ingredients to have a smoothened soup instead of broth.

UC-related Tips:

- Do not use pepper, garlic powder, and fresh parsley if you are experiencing a severe flare-up.

Nutrition Facts

Servings: 4

Amount per serving

Calories 127

	% Daily Value*
Total Fat 7.4g	9%
Saturated Fat 1.1g	6%
Cholesterol 0mg	0%
Sodium 1038mg	45%
Total Carbohydrate 14.9g	5%
Dietary Fiber 4.7g	17%
Total Sugars 7g	
Protein 1.8g	
Vitamin D 0mcg	0%
Calcium 90mg	7%
Iron 1mg	6%
Potassium 650mg	14%

HOMEMADE BEEF BROTH

An excellent idea for people living with UC to make their homemade beef broth instead of purchasing it from the stores. Many vegetable products are high in sodium and fat that are not good for Ulcerative Colitis patients. Beef broth is an excellent option for Ulcerative Colitis patients to consume when they are experiencing a flare-up.

- Prep Time: 10 minutes
- Cook Time: 60 minutes
- Total Time: 70 minutes
- Serving: 4-6

Ingredients

- 6 lbs organic grass-fed beef bones
- 2 celery stalks, chopped
- 3 carrots, chopped
- 3 bay leaves
- 1 teaspoon turmeric
- 1 tablespoon extra virgin olive oil
- 6 tablespoons apple cider vinegar
- 1 teaspoon dried thyme

132

- 2 tablespoons salt
- 1 teaspoon black pepper (optional)
- 1 teaspoon garlic powder (optional)

Instructions

1. Preheat oven to 400 °F.
2. Roast your bones, celery, carrots with extra virgin olive oil in the oven for 40 minutes.
3. At the same time, boil water and add bay leaves, apple cider vinegar, turmeric, thyme, salt, pepper, and garlic powder (optional) to it.
4. Add the roasted bones and vegetables to the water. Water should be enough to cover all ingredients.
5. Lid ajar and simmer all mix over slow heat for 20 minutes.
6. Remove all bones.
7. Clear the broth by a colander. Serve immediately or pour and store in a suitable bottle or jar for further use.

Cooking Tips:

- You can blend all ingredients to have a smoothened soup instead of broth, especially if you cooked meat pieces with bones.

UC-related Tips:

- Do not use pepper and garlic powder if you are experiencing a flare-up.

Nutrition Facts	
Servings: 4	
Amount per serving	
Calories	**122**
	% Daily Value*
Total Fat 5.2g	7%
Saturated Fat 2.1g	10%
Cholesterol 15mg	5%
Sodium 460mg	20%
Total Carbohydrate 14g	5%
Dietary Fiber 3.3g	12%
Total Sugars 4g	
Protein 9.6g	
Vitamin D 0mcg	0%
Calcium 37mg	3%
Iron 1mg	7%
Potassium 433mg	9%

RUSSIAN CHICKEN SOUP

A great, easy to cook Russian soup for cold winters. Great ingredients for Ulcerative Colitis patients!

- Prep Time: 10 minutes
- Cook Time: 30 minutes
- Total Time: 40 minutes
- Serving: 6

Ingredients

- 3 lbs organic, grass-fed chicken breasts, cubed 1 inch (~2.54 cm)
- ¾ cup Capellini or gluten-free pasta
- 4 cups low-sodium chicken or vegetable broth, or water
- 1 tablespoon extra virgin olive oil
- 1 carrot, skin-removed and cubed 1 inch (~2.54 cm)
- 4 medium potatoes, cubed & peeled 1 inch (~2.54 cm)
- 2 tablespoons fresh lemon juice
- 1 bay leaf
- Salt and pepper, to taste

- 1 teaspoon garlic powder (optional)

Instructions

1. Put all ingredients (except lemon juice and carrot) in a large pot and let it simmer over medium heat for 25 minutes.
2. Add carrots and lemon juice to the soup. Cook it for five more minutes. Then, adjust salt and pepper as desired.
3. Enjoy!

Cooking Tips:

- If you are in remission, you can fry chicken and carrot in a pan by one tablespoon of extra virgin olive oil and 1-teaspoon turmeric powder until golden brown. Then add chicken and carrot to the soup.

UC-related Tips:

- Do not use pepper and garlic powder if you are experiencing a flare-up.

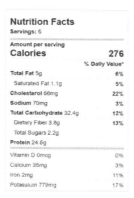

Nutrition Facts
Servings: 6

Amount per serving

Calories	276
	% Daily Value*
Total Fat 5g	6%
Saturated Fat 1.1g	5%
Cholesterol 66mg	22%
Sodium 70mg	3%
Total Carbohydrate 32.4g	12%
Dietary Fiber 3.8g	13%
Total Sugars 2.2g	
Protein 24.6g	
Vitamin D 0mcg	0%
Calcium 35mg	3%
Iron 2mg	11%
Potassium 779mg	17%

BABA GHANOUSH

A great vegetarian middle-eastern appetizer! You can serve Baba Ghanoush, hot or cold.

- Prep Time: 25 minutes
- Cook Time: 40 minutes
- Total Time: 65 minutes
- Serving: 4-6

<u>Ingredients</u>

- 2 eggplants, skin removed
- ¼ cup tahini
- 1 teaspoon extra virgin olive oil
- ½ tablespoon freshly squeezed lemon juice
- ¼ teaspoon salt
- ¼ teaspoon cumin powder
- 1 teaspoon garlic powder (optional)
- 1 tablespoon fresh parsley, chopped (optional)

<u>Instructions</u>

1. Place eggplants, cut thin lengthwise into a baking sheet with olive oil. Prick all surfaces with a fork. Broil all sides until it gets golden brown and smell smoky.
2. Turn off the broiler. Heat eggplants in the oven in a 375 °F. Let the eggplants roast for 30 minutes.
3. Remove eggplants from the oven. Cool down for 10 minutes and then add the tahini, lemon juice, garlic powder (optional), cumin powder and salt to it.
4. Mash the roasted mix with a fork until getting a great smooth texture.
5. Drizzle a little bit of olive oil and fresh parsley on top. Enjoy!

<u>Cooking Tips:</u>

- You can use roasted zucchini instead of the eggplants as well.

<u>UC-related Tips:</u>

- Do not use pepper and garlic powder if you are experiencing a severe flare-up.
- It is better to use the eggplants with no seeds/fewer seeds, especially if you have complications such as large intestinal strictures.

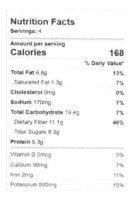

SALMON BRUSCHETTA

Experience great tastes of salmon, bread, and cheese!

- Prep Time: 10 minutes
- Cook Time: 30 minutes
- Total Time: 40 minutes
- Serving: 4

<u>Ingredients</u>

- ½ cup smoked salmon, thinly sliced
- 8 baguette slices or gluten-free bread/baguette

- ½ cup low-fat cream cheese or lactose-free cheese such as Swiss
- 1 tablespoon grated horseradish
- 1 tablespoon fresh lemon juice
- 1 tablespoon extra virgin olive oil
- 1 cup Persian cucumbers, peeled & chopped
- 1 teaspoon lemon zest

Instructions

1. Cut your baguette to have 1-inch (~2.54 cm) pieces. Then, toast your baguette pieces.
2. Mix cheese, horseradish, olive oil, lemon juice, and zest in a bowl. Grate cucumbers in it.
3. Spread your mix on toast slices and put smoked salmon on top. Enjoy!

Cooking Tips:

- You can use toasts instead of baguette to have a delicious cold sandwich.

Nutrition Facts

Servings: 4

Amount per serving

Calories	224
	% Daily Value*
Total Fat 14.8g	19%
Saturated Fat 7.2g	36%
Cholesterol 36mg	12%
Sodium 388mg	17%
Total Carbohydrate 14.9g	5%
Dietary Fiber 0.8g	3%
Total Sugars 1.1g	
Protein 8.2g	
Vitamin D 0mcg	0%
Calcium 38mg	3%
Iron 1mg	6%
Potassium 110mg	2%

GUACAMOLE-LIKE APPETIZER

A modified guacamole recipe for Ulcerative Colitis patients.

- Prep Time: 5 minutes
- Cook Time: 0 minutes
- Total Time: 5 minutes
- Serving: 4-6

Ingredients

- 6 avocados, peeled
- ½ tablespoon extra virgin olive oil
- ¼ cup chopped fresh cilantro
- 2 tablespoons fresh lime juice
- 1 teaspoon fresh lemon juice
- ½ teaspoon salt

Instructions

1- In a large bowl, mash avocados.
2- Add extra virgin olive oil and other ingredients into it.
3- Enjoy!

Cooking Tips:

- You can serve guacamole with tacos if you can tolerate it.
- If you can tolerate tomatoes and onions (in small amounts), cube, and add them into your guacamole.

UC-related Tips:

- Do not use fresh cilantro if you are experiencing a severe flare-up. Do not take taco chips, as well.

Nutrition Facts

Servings: 6

Amount per serving

Calories 422

	% Daily Value*
Total Fat 40.4g	52%
Saturated Fat 8.4g	42%
Cholesterol 0mg	0%
Sodium 207mg	9%
Total Carbohydrate 18g	7%
Dietary Fiber 13.5g	48%
Total Sugars 1.2g	
Protein 3.9g	
Vitamin D 0mcg	0%
Calcium 26mg	2%
Iron 1mg	7%
Potassium 988mg	21%

HOMEMADE LEBANESE HUMMUS

A healthy and tasty middle-eastern appetizer. An excellent option for vegetarians and Ulcerative Colitis patients in remission.

- Prep Time: 5 minutes
- Cook Time: 60 minutes
- Total Time: 65 minutes
- Serving: 4

Ingredients

- ¼ lb dried chickpeas (soaked in water for one night)
- 1½ tablespoons tahini
- 1 tablespoon lemon juice
- 2 tablespoons extra virgin olive oil, divided
- ¼ teaspoon cumin
- ½ teaspoon salt
- 1 tablespoon water
- 1 teaspoon baking soda (optional)
- 1 teaspoon paprika powder (optional)
- ½ teaspoon garlic powder (optional)

Instructions

1- First, Ulcerative Colitis patients need to soak the chickpeas overnight in water and optionally add baking soda to the water.
2- Cook your chickpeas in a large pot with water over medium heat for about 1 hour. Check if chickpeas cooked well by crushing one of them with a fork in your hand.
3- When chickpeas cooked, drain them and put them in a blender.
4- Add 1 tablespoon of extra virgin olive oil, lemon juice, tahini, cumin powder, salt, and garlic powder (optional) to the blender. Blend until your hummus gets a soft, creamy texture equally.
5- Sprinkle with 1 tablespoon extra virgin olive oil or paprika powder (optional).
6- Serve immediately or fridge it.

Cooking Tips:

- Hummus is well-matched with white pita bread.
- You can serve hummus, hot or cold.

UC-related Tips:

- Do not use paprika and garlic powders in hummus if you are experiencing a severe flare-up.
- Eat hummus in moderation when you are in remission. During a flare-up, it is better not to make this recipe or make and consume in a small amount.

Nutrition Facts

Servings: 4

Amount per serving

Calories 198

% Daily Value*

Total Fat 11.8g	15%
Saturated Fat 1.6g	8%
Cholesterol 0mg	0%
Sodium 305mg	13%
Total Carbohydrate 18.5g	7%
Dietary Fiber 5.5g	20%
Total Sugars 3.1g	
Protein 6.5g	
Vitamin D 0mcg	0%
Calcium 56mg	4%
Iron 2mg	13%
Potassium 279mg	6%

CRAB DIP WITH WONTON CHIPS

A great, easy-to-make appetizer with crabs in wonton wrappers!

- Prep Time: 5 minutes
- Cook Time: 30 minutes
- Total Time: 35 minutes
- Serving: 6

<u>Ingredients</u>

- 1 package Wonton wrappers or gluten-free wonton wrappers
- 1 teaspoon extra virgin olive oil
- 1 can crab meat, chopped
- ½ cup organic mayonnaise
- 1 tablespoon soy sauce
- ½ cup cream cheese or lactose-free cheese
- ½ teaspoon lemon juice
- 1 scallion, chopped
- 1 tablespoon honey or maple syrup
- 1 teaspoon salt, divided
- ½ teaspoon garlic powder (optional)

- ½ teaspoon black pepper (optional)

Instructions

1- Preheat oven to 400 °F.
2- Mix all ingredients into a large mixing bowl. Stir well.
3- In a baking dish, pour all the mix and bake for 30 minutes until you see edge bubbles.
4- Diagonally cut wonton wrappers in half and make triangles. Alternatively, you can make wonton cups.
5- Pour the cups with your mix.
6- Spray extra virgin olive oil on a baking sheet. Put triangles on it and spray olive oil on wontons as well. Add salt as desired. Let the wontons bake for 7 minutes until golden brown.
7- Remove from the oven. Serve and Enjoy!

Cooking Tips:

- You need to watch wontons while baking carefully. They can be burnt fast.
- You can have one teaspoon of stevia instead of honey or maple syrup if you cannot tolerate them.

UC-related Tips:

- Do not use pepper and garlic powders if you are experiencing a severe flare-up.
- When during a flare-up, boil scallion first and then add it to the mix.

Nutrition Facts	
Servings: 6	
Amount per serving	
Calories	**223**
	% Daily Value*
Total Fat 14.5g	19%
Saturated Fat 5.4g	27%
Cholesterol 46mg	15%
Sodium 881mg	38%
Total Carbohydrate 18.2g	6%
Dietary Fiber 0.3g	1%
Total Sugars 4.3g	
Protein 7.5g	
Vitamin D 0mcg	0%
Calcium 48mg	4%
Iron 1mg	6%
Potassium 128mg	3%

SHRIMP SALAD

Are you looking for a delicious salad with shrimp? You can follow this recipe to have one!

- Prep Time: 5 minutes
- Cook Time: 15 minutes
- Total Time: 20 minutes
- Serving: 2-4

Ingredients

- 1 lb shrimp, peeled
- 1 celery stalk, chopped
- 1 tablespoon extra virgin olive oil
- 1 tablespoon fresh lemon juice
- 1 teaspoon Dijon mustard
- ½ teaspoon turmeric powder
- Salt and pepper, to taste
- 2 tablespoons organic low-fat mayonnaise (optional)

Instructions

1. Cook shrimps by extra virgin olive oil and turmeric in a medium pan over medium heat.

2. In a large bowl, mix all lemon juice, Dijon mustard, salt, pepper, and mayonnaise (optional).
3. Add cooked shrimp to the bowl and combine.
4. Serve and enjoy!

Cooking Tips:

- You can prepare your shrimps in the oven as well. Just preheat oven to 375 °F. Choose a cooking sheet and spray olive oil on it. Put shrimp on your cooking sheet and let it cook until golden brown (around 10 minutes).
- You can add cubed pickles into your sauce mix to enjoy your shrimps with a great Tartar sauce.

UC-related Tips:

- Do not use pepper and mayonnaise if you are experiencing a flare-up. Use mustard in moderation as well.

Nutrition Facts

Servings: 4

Amount per serving

Calories	197
	% Daily Value*
Total Fat 8g	10%
Saturated Fat 1.5g	7%
Cholesterol 241mg	80%
Sodium 347mg	15%
Total Carbohydrate 3.9g	1%
Dietary Fiber 0.2g	1%
Total Sugars 0.6g	
Protein 26g	
Vitamin D 0mcg	0%
Calcium 107mg	8%
Iron 1mg	3%
Potassium 217mg	5%

ZUCCHINI SALAD (SPIRALIZED)

A great summer salad based on a zucchini. Zucchini salad is a healthy choice for Ulcerative Colitis patients.

- Prep Time: 30 minutes
- Total Time: 30 minutes
- Serving: 2-4

Ingredients

- 2 zucchinis, chopped
- ¼ cup low-fat/fat-free feta cheese or lactose-free aged cheddar
- 1 tablespoon extra virgin olive oil
- 2 tablespoons fresh lemon juice
- 1 tablespoon parsley, chopped (optional)
- Salt and pepper, to taste

Instructions

1. Make spiral zucchinis or cut them thin and lengthwise
2. In a large bowl, mix zucchinis and all other ingredients.
3. For better taste, let it rest for 15 minutes. Enjoy!

Cooking Tips:

- You can use vegetable peelers if you do not have a spiralizer.

UC-related Tips:

- Do not use pepper if you are experiencing a severe flare-up.
- Check if you can tolerate fresh parsley well or not. If you cannot tolerate, remove it from the recipe.

Nutrition Facts

Servings: 4

Amount per serving

Calories **65**

	% Daily Value*
Total Fat 3.7g	5%
Saturated Fat 0.6g	3%
Cholesterol 2mg	1%
Sodium 141mg	6%
Total Carbohydrate 3.9g	1%
Dietary Fiber 1.1g	4%
Total Sugars 1.9g	
Protein 4.8g	
Vitamin D 0mcg	0%
Calcium 65mg	5%
Iron 0mg	2%
Potassium 266mg	6%

OLIVIER SALAD (CHICKEN, POTATO & EGG SALAD)

A traditional well-known Russian salad with great ingredients for Ulcerative Colitis patients. For having a better taste, you can refrigerate it for 30 minutes.

- Prep Time: 15 minutes
- Cook Time: 45 minutes
- Total Time: 60 minutes
- Serving: 6

Ingredients

- 4 potatoes, skin removed and chopped
- 2 cups chicken breasts, shredded
- 2 organic, free-range eggs
- 2 medium carrots
- 4 dill pickles, cubed
- 2 tablespoons extra virgin olive oil
- 2 tablespoons fresh lemon juice
- 1 cup organic low-fat mayonnaise
- Salt and pepper, to taste

Instructions

1. Cook eggs, potatoes, and carrots in a large pot over medium/high heat. Use enough water to cover all ingredients.
2. Mash potatoes and eggs. Cube carrots and pickles (0.3-inch size).
3. In a large bowl, mix all ingredients well.
4. Refrigerate it for 10-15 minutes. Enjoy!

Cooking Tips:

- You can cube your potatoes and eggs similar to carrots, instead of mashing them.

UC-related Tips:

- Do not use pepper and mayonnaise if you are experiencing a flare-up.
- Always use mayo in moderation. If you cannot tolerate, use plain yogurt or lactose-free plain yogurt.

Nutrition Facts

Servings: 6

Amount per serving

Calories 300

	% Daily Value*
Total Fat 10.2g	13%
Saturated Fat 2.2g	11%
Cholesterol 111mg	37%
Sodium 931mg	40%
Total Carbohydrate 28.6g	10%
Dietary Fiber 4.4g	16%
Total Sugars 5.5g	
Protein 23.8g	
Vitamin D 5mcg	26%
Calcium 40mg	3%
Iron 2mg	11%
Potassium 756mg	16%

APPLE-PEAR SALAD WITH A SPECIAL VINAIGRETTE

A simple great fruit salad for everyone!

- Prep Time: 10 minutes

- Total Time: 10 minutes
- Serving: 4-6

Ingredients

- 3 cooked pears, peeled and chopped
- 1 papaya, peeled and chopped
- 3 apples, peeled and chopped
- ¼ cup honey or maple syrup
- 3 tablespoons fresh lemon juice
- ¼ cup fresh mint leaves, chopped (optional)

Instructions

1. Add all your ingredients in a large bowl and mix well.
2. Serve cold. Enjoy!

Cooking Tips:

- You can add ½ cup of other fruits like pineapple or peach if you can tolerate it.
- Remove honey or maple syrup from ingredients if you cannot tolerate any of them.

UC-related Tips:

- Check if you can tolerate fresh mint leaves or not. Remove from ingredients if you cannot tolerate it.

Nutrition Facts	
Servings: 4	
Amount per serving	
Calories	**278**
	% Daily Value*
Total Fat 0.8g	1%
Saturated Fat 0.1g	1%
Cholesterol 0mg	0%
Sodium 13mg	1%
Total Carbohydrate 73.2g	27%
Dietary Fiber 10.4g	37%
Total Sugars 56.5g	
Protein 1.6g	
Vitamin D 0mcg	0%
Calcium 33mg	3%
Iron 1mg	7%
Potassium 529mg	11%

BEET, CARROT & APPLE SALAD

A colorful salad with amazing fruits and vegetables inside!

- Prep Time: 10 minutes
- Total Time: 10 minutes
- Serving: 4-6

Ingredients

- 1 lb beet, peeled and cubed 1 inch (~2.54 cm)
- 2 medium carrots, peeled and cubed 1 inch (~2.54 cm)
- 1 apple, peeled and cubed 1 inch (~2.54 cm)
- 3 tablespoons fresh orange juice
- 2 tablespoons fresh lime juice
- 1 tablespoon extra virgin olive oil
- Salt and pepper, to taste
- ¼ cup fresh mint leaves, chopped (optional)

Instructions

1. In a large bowl, mix well all ingredients.
2. Serve cold. Enjoy!

Cooking Tips:

- You can add two tablespoons of balsamic vinegar if your gut can tolerate it.
- Wear gloves to cover your hands when you cut beets.

UC-related Tips:

- Check if you can tolerate fresh mint leaves or not. Remove from ingredients if you cannot tolerate it.
- Do not use pepper if you are experiencing a severe flare-up.
- Cook beets or remove it from ingredients when you are experiencing a flare-up.

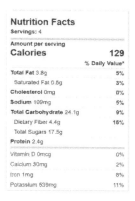

BUTTER LETTUCE SALAD WITH HONEY VINAIGRETTE

A light and delicious salad for Ulcerative Colitis patients who can tolerate butter lettuce with a delicious dressing.

- Prep Time: 15 minutes
- Total Time: 15 minutes
- Serving: 4-6

Ingredients

- 2 medium butter lettuces, cut into small pieces (also called Bibb, Boston or living lettuce)
- 1 tablespoon honey or maple syrup
- 1 teaspoon Dijon mustard
- 2 tablespoons fresh lemon juice
- 2 tablespoons fresh lime juice
- 2 tablespoons extra virgin olive oil
- Salt and pepper to taste

Instructions

1. Wash butter lettuce thoroughly and cut into small pieces
2. In a large bowl, mix well all ingredients.
3. Serve cold. Enjoy!

Cooking Tips:

- You can add two peeled Persian cucumbers to have a garden-like salad!
- You can add one tablespoon of balsamic vinegar if your gut can tolerate it.

UC-related Tips:

- Butter lettuce, also called Bibb, living or Boston lettuce, is a type of lettuce that can be digested easier than other types of lettuce. Hence, it is an excellent option for Ulcerative Colitis patients to try butter lettuce and check if they can tolerate it or not. Many of Ulcerative Colitis patients can enjoy a garden salad with butter lettuce during remissions.
- Do not use pepper if you are experiencing a severe flare-up.

Nutrition Facts

Servings: 4

Amount per serving

Calories 91

	% Daily Value*
Total Fat 7.1g	9%
Saturated Fat 1.1g	5%
Cholesterol 0mg	0%
Sodium 21mg	1%
Total Carbohydrate 7.5g	3%
Dietary Fiber 1.1g	4%
Total Sugars 5.7g	
Protein 1.2g	
Vitamin D 0mcg	0%
Calcium 33mg	3%
Iron 0mg	1%
Potassium 237mg	5%

CARROT-AVOCADO SALAD

An epic salad recipe with avocado and tasty dressing. A great salad option for Ulcerative Colitis patients!

- Prep Time: 20 minutes
- Cook Time: 30 minutes
- Total Time: 50 minutes
- Serving: 4-6

Ingredients

- 1 large avocado
- 2 carrots, peeled and diced 1-inch (~2.54 cm)
- 2 tablespoons extra virgin olive oil
- 1 tablespoon fresh lemon juice
- Salt and pepper, to taste
- ⅓ cup green onion, chopped (optional)
- ¼ cup fresh mint leaves, chopped (optional)

Instructions

1. Peel-off carrots.
2. In a small pot, cook carrots in boiling water over medium heat.

3. Cube carrots and avocados. In a medium bowl, mix other ingredients and then add carrot and avocado.
4. Mix well. Enjoy!

Cooking Tips:

- You can cook carrots in a small pan with one tablespoon of extra virgin olive oil and ½ teaspoon of turmeric powder over medium heat as well.

UC-related Tips:

- Make sure your gut can tolerate green onion before using it.
- Do not use pepper, green onion, and fresh mint if you are experiencing a flare-up.

Nutrition Facts

Servings: 4

Amount per serving

Calories	179
	% Daily Value*
Total Fat 16.9g	22%
Saturated Fat 3.1g	15%
Cholesterol 0mg	0%
Sodium 26mg	1%
Total Carbohydrate 8g	3%
Dietary Fiber 4.4g	16%
Total Sugars 2g	
Protein 1.4g	
Vitamin D 0mcg	0%
Calcium 22mg	2%
Iron 1mg	3%
Potassium 369mg	8%

CLASSIC TUNA PASTA SALAD

Classic tuna with pasta is an excellent choice as your salad. You can have it for lunch or dinner as well.

- Prep Time: 15 minutes
- Cook Time: 15 minutes
- Total Time: 30 minutes

- Serving: 4

Ingredients

- 1½ cups pasta (rotini preferred), or gluten-free pasta
- 1 celery stalk, chopped
- 1 can tuna in water
- ½ cup organic low-fat mayonnaise
- ½ tablespoon ketchup (optional)
- 2 tablespoons white vinegar
- Salt and pepper, to taste

Instructions

1. Cook pasta according to its package instruction.
2. Drain pasta and place it in a large bowl.
3. Add celery, tuna, and all other ingredients to the pasta bowl. Mix well.
4. It is better to let it cool in the fridge for 30 minutes. Enjoy!

Cooking Tips:

- Instead of white vinegar, you can use one tablespoon of fresh lemon juice or one tablespoon sour grape juice.

UC-related Tips:

- Make sure your gut can tolerate ketchup before using it.
- Do not use pepper if you are experiencing a flare-up.

Nutrition Facts

Servings: 4

Amount per serving

Calories 105

	% Daily Value*
Total Fat 3g	4%
Saturated Fat 0.7g	3%
Cholesterol 25mg	8%
Sodium 526mg	23%
Total Carbohydrate 8.9g	3%
Dietary Fiber 1.4g	5%
Total Sugars 4.9g	
Protein 10.4g	
Vitamin D 0mcg	0%
Calcium 13mg	1%
Iron 1mg	3%
Potassium 159mg	3%

SALMON CEVICHE

This salad is full of omega-3 with a fabulous dressing. Enjoy this dairy-free, egg-free, nut-free, and gluten-free recipe.

- Prep Time: 15 minutes
- Rest Time: 15 minutes
- Total Time: 30 minutes
- Serving: 4

Ingredients

- 1 lb salmon, skin removed and cubed
- 1 cup Persian cucumber, cubed 1cm
- ½ cup green onion, chopped well
- 1 tablespoon fresh lemon juice
- 1 tablespoon fresh lime juice
- 1 tablespoon grated fresh ginger
- Salt and pepper, to taste
- 1 teaspoon dried oregano (optional)

Instructions

1. In a large bowl, mix salmon, cucumber, green onion, ginger, and oregano.
2. In a small cup/bowl, whisk lime & lemon juice, salt, and pepper and pour it into the large bowl.
3. Mix all well. Serve cold. Enjoy!

Cooking Tips:

- You can add ½ teaspoon freshly grated turmeric if you want to enjoy its anti-inflammatory properties.

UC-related Tips:

- Make sure your gut can tolerate green onion and oregano before using them.
- Do not use pepper if you are experiencing a flare-up.

Nutrition Facts

Servings: 4

Amount per serving

Calories	167
	% Daily Value*
Total Fat 7.1g	9%
Saturated Fat 1.1g	5%
Cholesterol 50mg	17%
Sodium 53mg	2%
Total Carbohydrate 3.9g	1%
Dietary Fiber 1.1g	4%
Total Sugars 0.6g	
Protein 22.4g	
Vitamin D 0mcg	0%
Calcium 52mg	4%
Iron 1mg	6%
Potassium 506mg	11%

HONEY MUSTARD CHICKEN SALAD

Enjoy making a rich salad with chicken and honey mustard. Excellent source of protein for Ulcerative Colitis patients.

- Prep Time: 25 minutes
- Total Time: 25 minutes

-   Serving: 4-6

Ingredients

- 1 lb chicken breasts, skinless and boneless
- 1 avocado, chopped
- 4 tablespoons honey or maple syrup
- 6 cups butter lettuce, chopped
- 3 tablespoons apple cider vinegar
- 2 tablespoons Dijon mustard
- 1 tablespoon low-fat feta cheese or lactose-free aged cheddar
- 2 tablespoons extra virgin olive oil
- Salt and pepper, to taste
- ½ teaspoon garlic powder (optional)
- 1 tablespoon green onion, chopped (optional)

Instructions

1. In a large pan, cook chickens with two tablespoons of extra virgin olive oil over medium heat until getting close to a golden brown. Remove from pan and cut into 1-inch (~2.54 cm) cubes.
2. In a large bowl, whisk honey (or maple syrup), mustard, vinegar, garlic powder (optional), green onion (optional), cheese, salt, and pepper.
3. In another large bowl, cut lettuce into small pieces. Add cubed chickens and pour the sauce on top. Serve and enjoy!

Cooking Tips:

- You can boil chickens in a pot over medium heat (recommended for flare-up times).

- If you cannot tolerate honey, use maple syrup or agave syrup instead.

UC-related Tips:

- Make sure your gut can tolerate green onion before using it.
- Do not use pepper and garlic powder if you are experiencing a flare-up.

Nutrition Facts

Servings: 0

Amount per serving

Calories	310
	% Daily Value*
Total Fat 17.1g	22%
Saturated Fat 3.6g	18%
Cholesterol 68mg	23%
Sodium 152mg	7%
Total Carbohydrate 16.5g	6%
Dietary Fiber 2.8g	10%
Total Sugars 12.3g	
Protein 23.6g	
Vitamin D 0mcg	0%
Calcium 29mg	2%
Iron 3mg	15%
Potassium 444mg	9%

MAIN COURSES

MEDITERRANEAN CHICKEN - ZUCCHINI STEW

Chicken – Zucchini stew is one of the delicious Mediterranean stews, which typically serves with steamed white rice. Turmeric, zucchini, and white rice are great for Ulcerative Colitis patients, and most can well-tolerate them.

- Prep Time: 10 minutes
- Cook Time: 50 minutes
- Total Time: 60 minutes
- Serving: 4

Ingredients

- 4 Fresh zucchinis, lengthwise-cut with no skin
- 6 Skin-removed chicken legs
- 4 tablespoons extra virgin olive oil
- 1.5 teaspoon turmeric
- ½ teaspoon black pepper
- 1½ teaspoons salt
- 3 tablespoons lemon juice or 1 lime
- 2½ cups water
- 4 tablespoons tomato paste (optional)

Preparation

1. Fry, both sides of skinless zucchinis with two tablespoons of extra virgin olive oil in a sauté pan until golden brown.
2. In another pan, fry your chicken legs with the rest of extra virgin olive oil, salt, pepper, and turmeric until golden brown.
3. Boil water in a pot and dissolve tomato paste to the boiling water if you want (optional). Stir well.
4. Add your chicken legs to the boiling water. Turn the heat to medium. Let it simmer for 20 minutes. If your sauce gets thick, add more water to your stew.
5. After 25 minutes, add your zucchinis and your lemon juice to the stew and let it cook for another 5 minutes. After three minutes, taste your stew and correct your seasonings. Do not add more black peppers.
6. Enjoy this meal with steamed white rice!

Cooking Tips:

- To reach a faster cooking time, you can add all the ingredients into the boiling water and let the stew cook for 40 minutes on high heat.

- You can use eggplant instead of zucchini to make a delicious Eggplant Stew. Just remember not to use the eggplants seeds or remove eggplant small edible seeds.

UC-related Tips:

- Some Ulcerative Colitis patients cannot tolerate tomato pastes. In that case, cook this stew without tomato paste or use two cups of organic beef bone broth instead of water.
- If you are in a flare-up, try not to use pepper and remove zucchini's skins.
- If you have a colon stricture, try not to alternate zucchini with eggplant with lots of seeds.

Nutrition Facts	
Servings: 4	
Amount per serving	
Calories	**352**
	% Daily Value*
Total Fat 22.6g	29%
Saturated Fat 4.4g	22%
Cholesterol 89mg	30%
Sodium 1001mg	44%
Total Carbohydrate 10.5g	4%
Dietary Fiber 3.1g	11%
Total Sugars 5.8g	
Protein 28.9g	
Vitamin D 0mcg	0%
Calcium 55mg	4%
Iron 3mg	16%
Potassium 945mg	20%

LACTOSE-FREE CHICKEN FETTUCCINE ALFREDO

Do you love to have a creamy-but-healthy Fettuccine Alfredo? You can use this recipe to have a delicious Italian main course. This meal has chicken/vegetable stock, turmeric, ginger, and lemon that are great for Ulcerative Colitis patients.

- Prep Time: 15 minutes

- Cook Time: 30 minutes
- Total Time: 45 minutes
- Serving: 4

Ingredients

- 4 boneless, skinless chicken breasts, about 0.8 inches (~2 cm) thick
- ¾ lb uncooked fettuccine (~340 g) or gluten-free fettuccine/pasta
- 3 tablespoons all-purpose flour or gluten-free flour
- 10 oz lactose-free milk (~300 ml)
- ½ cup unsalted organic chicken stock or vegetable stock (~120 ml)
- 1 tablespoon fresh lemon juice
- 3½ teaspoons Himalayan salt, divided
- 2 teaspoons black pepper, divided
- 1 teaspoon turmeric
- 1 teaspoon ginger powder
- 3 tablespoons extra virgin olive oil, divided
- 1 teaspoon garlic powder (optional)
- Fresh parsley, minced (optional)

Preparation

1. Heat a tablespoon of extra virgin olive oil in a pan. Add your chicken breast with one tablespoon of salt, one tablespoon of pepper and turmeric and let it cook for 5 minutes until golden brown both sides.
2. Boil the water in a large pot over high heat. Add one tablespoon of high-quality extra virgin olive oil and one tablespoon of salt to the water. Then, add your fettuccine in the boiling water.

3. Cook fettuccine according to its package instructions. Drain and return to the pot.
4. In another pan, put one tablespoon of extra virgin olive oil on medium heat. When heated, add your flour slowly and whisk until golden brown.
5. Heat your lactose-free milk in the microwave, add it slowly to your flour, and whisk for 3 minutes. Add lemon juice, ginger powder, garlic powder (optional), one tablespoon of pepper, and one tablespoon of salt to make an excellent béchamel sauce.
6. Add chicken/vegetable stock to the béchamel sauce, frequently stir for 10 minutes until thickened.
7. Slice or cube chicken. Add the béchamel sauce to your fettuccine pot and toss perfectly.
8. Garnish the top with minced parsley and enjoy!

Cooking Tips:

- If you are not lactose-intolerant, you can use regular cow milk.
- Béchamel sauce can be made with coconut milk, as well.
- If you are gluten intolerant, you can use gluten-free pasta/fettuccine.

UC-related Tips:

- Do not use garlic powder or parsley if you cannot tolerate it.
- Make sure that your chickens are skinless.
- If you are in a flare-up, try not to use pepper.

Nutrition Facts

Servings: 4

Amount per serving

Calories   **626**

	% Daily Value*
Total Fat 23.2g	30%
Saturated Fat 5.1g	25%
Cholesterol 170mg	57%
Sodium 2433mg	106%
Total Carbohydrate 51g	19%
Dietary Fiber 3.6g	13%
Total Sugars 1.3g	
Protein 50.5g	
Vitamin D 0mcg	0%
Calcium 52mg	4%
Iron 4mg	20%
Potassium 387mg	8%

CHICKEN WITH MASHED POTATOES

For those who want a very simple but delicious main course. Cooked baby carrot can be used as a well-matched garnish.

- Prep Time: 5 minutes
- Cook Time: 20 minutes
- Total Time: 25 minutes
- Serving: 4

Ingredients

- 4 skinless, boneless chicken breast
- 2 tablespoons extra virgin olive oil, divided
- 1½ cups unsalted chicken stock (organic preferred)
- 2 skin-removed large potatoes
- ½ cup lactose-free milk
- 1 teaspoon black pepper, divided
- ¼ teaspoon salt, divided
- ¼ teaspoon turmeric
- 1 tablespoon minced parsley (optional)

Preparation

1. High-heat 2 tablespoons of extra virgin olive oil in a pan. Add your chicken breast with ½ tablespoon of salt, pepper, and one tablespoon of turmeric and let it cook until golden brown both sides.
2. Cook all potatoes in a medium pot with a little pinch of turmeric.
3. Mash your potatoes and add the rest of salt and pepper.
4. Heat lactose-free milk in the microwave and add to your mashed potato. Whisk well.
5. Pour your plate with mashed potato, and chicken on top.

Cooking Tips:

- If you are not lactose-intolerant, you can use low-fat normal cow whole milk.
- You can make the Béchamel sauce (explained before in Fettuccine Alfredo recipe) and add it to your chicken and mashed potato.

UC-related Tips:

- Do not use parsley if you cannot tolerate it.
- Make sure that your chickens and potatoes are skinless as Ulcerative Colitis patients may not tolerate skins
- If you are in a flare-up, try not to use pepper.

Nutrition Facts		
Servings: 4		
Amount per serving		
Calories		448
		% Daily Value*
Total Fat 15.8g		20%
Saturated Fat 3.1g		16%
Cholesterol 108mg		36%
Sodium 279mg		12%
Total Carbohydrate 33g		12%
Dietary Fiber 3.3g		12%
Total Sugars 3.1g		
Protein 42.8g		
Vitamin D 0mcg		0%
Calcium 49mg		4%
Iron 3mg		14%
Potassium 911mg		19%

CHICKEN STROGANOFF

Try Chicken Stroganoff with potatoes and incredible gravy, matched with Ulcerative Colitis patient tolerance levels.

- Prep Time: 5 minutes
- Cook Time: 15 minutes
- Total Time: 20 minutes
- Serving: 4

Ingredients

- 4 skinless, boneless chicken breast
- 2 tablespoons all-purpose flour or gluten-free flour
- 2 cups (~500 ml) unsalted/salt-reduced beef broth (organic preferred)
- 1 tablespoon of salt and pepper
- 3 tablespoons extra virgin olive oil
- 1 tablespoon Dijon mustard
- ⅓ cup lactose-free milk
- 1 tablespoon fresh lemon juice
- ½ tablespoon ginger powder or fresh ginger
- ½ tablespoon turmeric

- 10 oz (~300 gr) mushrooms, thickly sliced
- ½ tsp garlic powder (optional)
- Parsley, minced (optional)

Instructions

1. Heat a tablespoon of high-quality extra virgin olive oil in a pan. Flat your chicken breasts and cook them with ½ tablespoon of salt, ½ tablespoon of pepper and ginger powder until golden brown both sides.
2. In another pan, put one tablespoon of extra virgin olive oil on medium heat. When heated, sauté your mushrooms. Then, add your flour slowly and whisk until golden brown.
3. Heat your lactose-free milk in the microwave, add it slowly to your flour, and whisk for 3 minutes. Add lemon juice, garlic powder (optional), Dijon mustard, ½ tablespoon of pepper, and ½ tablespoon of salt to make a great sauce. Stir the sauce on low heat until it becomes thick.
4. Fry very thin-sliced potatoes with one tablespoon of extra virgin olive oil and ½ tablespoon of turmeric.
5. Add your fries and chicken to your sauce. Let it cook for two more minutes.
6. Garnish the top with minced parsley and enjoy!

Cooking Tips:

- If you are not lactose-intolerant, you can use low-fat cow whole milk.
- You can use pork tenderloin or turkey breast instead of chicken breast.
- If you like, you can serve it with any pasta as well.

UC-related Tips:

- Make sure that your chickens and potatoes are skinless as Ulcerative Colitis patients may not tolerate skins.
- If you are in a flare-up, try not to use pepper.
- If you are in a flare-up, try to Airfry your fries or boil them.
- Do not use mushrooms or parsley if you cannot tolerate them.

Nutrition Facts

Servings: 4

Amount per serving

Calories	274
	% Daily Value*
Total Fat 13.2g	17%
Saturated Fat 1.9g	10%
Cholesterol 67mg	22%
Sodium 433mg	19%
Total Carbohydrate 10.7g	4%
Dietary Fiber 2.6g	9%
Total Sugars 2.7g	
Protein 29.8g	
Vitamin D 15mcg	77%
Calcium 42mg	3%
Iron 3mg	17%
Potassium 331mg	7%

CHICKEN KEBAB

Enjoy a classic barbecued chicken, well-marinated in saffron and yogurt!

- Prep Time: 15 minutes
- (Marinate Time: 2 hours)
- Cook Time: 25 minutes
- Total Time: 40 minutes
- Serving: 4

Ingredients

- 4 chicken breasts, cut into 1.5 inches (3.8) cubes
- ¾ cup lactose-free yogurt or plain yogurt if you are not lactose intolerant

- 1 large onion
- ¼ cup saffron (bloomed)
- 1 tablespoon salt
- 3 tablespoons extra virgin olive oil
- 1 tablespoon lemon juice

Instructions

1. Cut your onions and make onion rings.
2. To marinate your chicken, mix and stir it well with onion, lactose-free plain yogurt, bloomed saffron, olive oil, salt, and lemon juice together (To have a bloomed saffron, you need to grind your saffron perfectly and add 100ml of boiling water to it).
3. Cover the marinated bowl and put it in the fridge to rest for two hours.
4. After two hours, thread chickens into skewers and grilled both sides well until golden brown

Cooking Tips:

- If you are not lactose-intolerant, you can use low-fat plain yogurt.
- You can use the oven instead of grilling chickens. Just preheat the oven to 400 °F, cover chickens with aluminum foils, and let it cook for about 25 minutes. Use broil for five minutes if you want a golden brown texture.
- You can use chicken with bones instead of chicken breasts, as well.

UC-related Tips:

- If you cannot tolerate saffron (rarely happens), do not add saffron to chicken. Instead, put ⅓ tablespoon of turmeric.

Nutrition Facts	
Servings: 4	
Amount per serving	
Calories	**322**
	% Daily Value*
Total Fat 21g	27%
Saturated Fat 2.5g	12%
Cholesterol 68mg	23%
Sodium 1812mg	79%
Total Carbohydrate 7.4g	3%
Dietary Fiber 0.9g	3%
Total Sugars 1.7g	
Protein 27.6g	
Vitamin D 0mcg	0%
Calcium 70mg	5%
Iron 0mg	2%
Potassium 174mg	4%

ROASTED CHICKEN WITH POMEGRANATE SAUCE

Have you tried a sour taste of chicken with pomegranate sauce? This dish is an excellent sample of a delicious sour chicken. You can make your dish sweet and sour by adding honey to the recipe.

- Prep Time: 10 minutes
- (Marinate Time: 2 hours)
- Cook Time: 40 minutes
- Total Time: 50 minutes
- Serving: 4

<u>Ingredients</u>

- 4 Chicken legs and thighs, skinless
- ¼ cup bloomed saffron
- 2 tablespoons extra virgin olive oil
- 5 tablespoons lime juice
- ½ cup pomegranate sauce
- 1 tablespoon salt

- 1 tablespoon turmeric
- 2 cups of water
- ½ tablespoon Black pepper
- ½ cup honey (optional)

Instructions

1. In a large bowl, marinate your chicken with bloomed saffron, lime juice, honey (optional) salt and pepper.
2. Mix and stir all ingredients well. Cover the bowl top and fridge it for 2 hours.
3. Roast your chicken with extra virgin olive oil and turmeric for 15 minutes until golden brown.
4. Boil two cups of water and add pomegranate sauce. Stir well until dissolved.
5. Put your chicken in the sauce and let it cook for 25 minutes. Let the sauce thicken, and then you are done!
6. Serve it with white basmati rice and enjoy!

Cooking Tips:

- Alternatively, you may want to use chicken breasts instead of chicken legs and thighs.
- If you do not find the pomegranate sauce or paste, you can add 200ml of pomegranate juice. It makes your meal hard to be thickened, but it gives you a similar taste.

UC-related Tips:

- If you cannot tolerate saffron (rarely happens), do not add saffron to chicken. Instead, put ⅓ tablespoon of turmeric.

- Pomegranate has anti-inflammatory properties, which is excellent for Ulcerative Colitis patients, and it can be well-tolerate in many patients. However, if you cannot tolerate it, use dark grape juice instead. Make sure pomegranates are consumed seedless.

Nutrition Facts

Servings: 4

Amount per serving

Calories 303

	% Daily Value*
Total Fat 17.2g	22%
Saturated Fat 3.6g	18%
Cholesterol 90mg	30%
Sodium 2084mg	91%
Total Carbohydrate 16.4g	6%
Dietary Fiber 0.6g	2%
Total Sugars 11.4g	
Protein 22.7g	
Vitamin D 0mcg	0%
Calcium 33mg	3%
Iron 2mg	13%
Potassium 79mg	2%

PUFFY CHICKEN

A tremendous yummy puffy chicken strips for adults and kids.

- Prep Time: 10 minutes
- Cook Time: 20 minutes
- Total Time: 30 minutes
- Serving: 4

Ingredients

- 4 strip cuts of chicken breast (~400 grams)
- 150 grams of all-purpose flour or gluten-free flour
- 5 tablespoons alcohol-free carbonated malt drink
- 2 tablespoons extra virgin olive oil
- 3 eggs (organic range-free preferred)
- 1 tablespoon Dijon mustard
- ½ tablespoon salt

- ½ tablespoon turmeric powder
- ½ teaspoon stevia or maple syrup (optional)
- 1 tablespoon active dried yeast (optional)

Instructions

1. In a large bowl, marinate your chicken with malt drink, yeast, olive oil, mustard, salt, and turmeric. Mix all well.
2. In another bowl, whisk all three eggs perfectly.
3. First, deep your marinated chickens into eggs and then cover it with flour.
4. Cook your chicken in a pan over medium heat with extra virgin olive oil.

Cooking Tips:

- You can use stevia or maple syrup to give a sweet taste to your dish.
- Instead of carbonated malt drink, you can use carbonated water. In this case, you need to use active dry yeast.

UC-related Tips:

- If you are in a flare-up, put your marinated chicken in boiling water instead of frying it.
- If you can tolerate beer a little bit, you can use it instead of malt drink.
- This dish is well-matched with Tartar sauce. So, if you tolerate Tartar, enjoy this meal with it!

Nutrition Facts
Servings: 4

Amount per serving

Calories   **458**

	% Daily Value*
Total Fat 16g	20%
Saturated Fat 3.5g	18%
Cholesterol 221mg	74%
Sodium 1061mg	46%
Total Carbohydrate 31.8g	12%
Dietary Fiber 1.3g	5%
Total Sugars 2g	
Protein 44.3g	
Vitamin D 12mcg	58%
Calcium 46mg	4%
Iron 4mg	22%
Potassium 410mg	9%

CHICKEN SCALOPPINI

Enjoy a delicious Italian dish with ingredients great for Ulcerative Colitis patients!

- Prep Time: 10 minutes
- Cook Time: 15 minutes
- Total Time: 25 minutes
- Serving: 4

Ingredients

- 4 skinless and boneless chicken breast
- 2 teaspoons fresh lemon juice
- 1 tablespoon extra virgin olive oil
- 6 tablespoons bread crumbs or any gluten-free dried bread
- ½ cup unsalted, no-fat chicken broth
- 1 tablespoon lime juice
- 1 tablespoon well-cooked capers
- ¼ teaspoon salt
- ¼ teaspoon black pepper
- ¼ cup grape vinegar (optional)

Instructions

1. First, use a meat mallet to pound your chicken breasts.
2. Add lemon juice, salt, and pepper to your chicken
3. Heat a pan with extra virgin olive oil over medium heat. Add your chicken to the pan and cook each side for about 5 minutes until golden brown.
4. In the end, add chicken broth, grape vinegar (optional), and your breadcrumbs and stir well for five more minutes until it gets thick.
5. Garnish with capers. Enjoy!

Cooking Tips:

- You can use sour grape juice or grape vinegar if you want to give a bitter taste to your meal.

UC-related Tips:

- If you can tolerate sour grape juice or grape vinegar, you can add it to your broth.
- Make sure you cooked capers well.
- Just use peppers if you can tolerate them.
- If you are in a flare-up, do not need to fry chicken. Just boil it in chicken broth.

Nutrition Facts

Servings: 4

Amount per serving

Calories	**320**

% Daily Value*

Total Fat 11g	14%
Saturated Fat 2.6g	13%
Cholesterol 35mg	12%
Sodium 863mg	38%
Total Carbohydrate 33.2g	12%
Dietary Fiber 1.5g	6%
Total Sugars 0.7g	
Protein 20.8g	
Vitamin D 0mcg	0%
Calcium 18mg	1%
Iron 2mg	9%
Potassium 28mg	1%

CHICKEN-PINEAPPLE PIZZA

Do you think lactose-intolerant Ulcerative Colitis patients cannot eat pizza anymore? You might be wrong! Try this recipe to have a great pizza taste!

- Prep Time: 10 minutes
- Cook Time: 15 minutes
- Total Time: 25 minutes
- Serving: 4

Ingredients

- 4 gluten-free pizza crusts
- 1 cup sliced no-fat cooked chicken breast
- 1 cup pineapple chunks
- 1 cup shredded mozzarella or lactose-free cheese
- 4 tablespoons organic mayonnaise
- 1 teaspoon oregano powder

Instructions

1. Place your gluten-free pizza crusts on a non-stick pizza pan or bake sheet.

2. Spread your organic low-fat low-sodium mayo on your crust.
3. Add your cooked chicken breasts and pineapple to your pizza
4. Sprinkle with mozzarella or lactose-free cheese
5. Let it bake at 480 °F for 10 minutes. Then, broil on the same heat for five more minutes until cheese melted.

Cooking Tips:

- You can use any other white sauces such as béchamel sauce instead of mayo.

UC-related Tips:

- If you are lactose intolerant, use lactose-free or dairy-free cheese for pizza
- Use mayonnaise only if you can tolerate it. If you cannot tolerate, you can make a béchamel sauce instead (explained before in Fettuccine Alfredo recipe).

Nutrition Facts	
Servings: 4	
Amount per serving	
Calories	**342**
	% Daily Value*
Total Fat 12.4g	16%
Saturated Fat 2.7g	14%
Cholesterol 47mg	16%
Sodium 499mg	22%
Total Carbohydrate 39.1g	14%
Dietary Fiber 2.1g	7%
Total Sugars 7g	
Protein 18.5g	
Vitamin D 0mcg	0%
Calcium 82mg	6%
Iron 1mg	7%
Potassium 165mg	4%

TURKEY ZUCCHINI NOODLES

If you look for a healthy meal for your lunch or dinner, you can try Turkey Zucchini Noodles. If you have some leftover turkeys from Thanksgiving or any other events, it would be an excellent option for you to cook this delicious main course.

- Prep Time: 15 minutes
- Cook Time: 15 minutes
- Total Time: 30 minutes
- Serving: 4

Ingredients

- 3 medium-size spiralized zucchinis or zucchini strips
- 1 lb (~455 g) skinless fat-free cooked turkey breasts
- 1 tablespoon extra virgin olive oil, divided
- 2 cups of water
- ½ teaspoon turmeric
- ½ teaspoon salt
- 1 tablespoon tomato paste (optional)
- ¼ teaspoon stevia (optional)

Instructions

1. Cook zucchini noodles in boiling water for 5 minutes.
2. Bring them out of the water and let them dry.
3. Heat your cooked turkey in a pan with extra virgin olive oil. Add turmeric, tomato paste (optional), stevia (optional) salt, and little water (~100ml) for 5 minutes until golden brown both sides.
4. Add your zucchini to your turkey and stir well. Enjoy!

Cooking Tips:

- You can use a can of organic crushed tomatoes instead of tomato paste if you can tolerate them.

<u>UC-related Tips:</u>

- If you are in a flare-up, do not need to golden-brown turkey. Just boil it in 1 cup of zucchini water.

Nutrition Facts
Servings: 4

Amount per serving

Calories	172
	% Daily Value*
Total Fat 5.7g	7%
Saturated Fat 0.9g	5%
Cholesterol 49mg	16%
Sodium 1460mg	63%
Total Carbohydrate 9.9g	4%
Dietary Fiber 2.3g	8%
Total Sugars 6.5g	
Protein 21.2g	
Vitamin D 0mcg	0%
Calcium 35mg	3%
Iron 2mg	13%
Potassium 736mg	16%

ZUCCHINI EGG DISH

Are you looking for a vegetarian dish that is well-matched with Ulcerative Colitis patient diet? Try a fabulous Zucchini Egg dish.

- Prep Time: 10 minutes
- Cook Time: 15 minutes
- Total Time: 25 minutes
- Serving: 4

<u>Ingredients</u>

- 3 medium-size, diced zucchinis
- 2 organic range-free eggs
- 1 tablespoon garlic powder
- 1 tablespoon extra virgin olive oil
- ½ teaspoon turmeric powder
- ½ teaspoon salt
- ½ teaspoon black pepper

Instructions

1. Peels off zucchinis and cook them in a pan over medium heat.
2. When zucchinis become soft, flattened them or blend them in a blender.
3. Add garlic powder, turmeric, salt, and pepper to your pan.
4. Whisk eggs in a small bowl and add them to your zucchinis.
5. When the eggs get coagulate, mix them with your zucchinis. Enjoy!

Cooking Tips:

- You can use eggplant instead of zucchini.
- You can also add one tablespoon of tomato paste if you can tolerate it.

UC-related Tips:

- If you are in a flare-up, do not need to fry zucchinis. Just boil them in 1 cup of water.
- Do not use black pepper in your meal if you are in a severe flare-up.

Nutrition Facts	
Servings: 4	
Amount per serving	
Calories	**94**
	% Daily Value*
Total Fat 6g	8%
Saturated Fat 1.2g	6%
Cholesterol 82mg	27%
Sodium 337mg	15%
Total Carbohydrate 7g	3%
Dietary Fiber 2g	7%
Total Sugars 3.2g	
Protein 5g	
Vitamin D 8mcg	39%
Calcium 37mg	3%
Iron 1mg	7%
Potassium 448mg	10%

POTATO CUTLET

Potato Cutlet is an easy to cook vegetarian recipe for Ulcerative Colitis patients with a yummy crispy texture.

- Prep Time: 10 minutes
- Cook Time: 20 minutes
- Total Time: 30 minutes
- Serving: 4

Ingredients

- 2 lbs yellow skin-removed potatoes
- 5 large organic range-free eggs
- 3 tablespoons extra virgin olive oil
- ½ teaspoon turmeric powder
- Salt and black pepper to taste

Instructions

1. Remove potato skins and scrub potatoes with a scrubber.
2. In a large bowl, mix potatoes and all other ingredients perfectly.
3. Make potato cutlets by rounding-and-flattening them in your hand.
4. Heat your high-quality extra virgin olive oil in a skillet over medium heat. Add your cutlets to the pan and flatten them.
5. Let it cook each side until golden brown.

Cooking Tips:

- You can add one teaspoon freshly grated ginger to your ingredients, as well.

UC-related Tips:

- If you are in a flare-up, do not need to fry potatoes. Just boil them in water and then mix them with other ingredients.
- Do not use black pepper in your meal if you are in a severe flare-up.

Nutrition Facts

Servings: 4

Amount per serving

Calories	273
	% Daily Value*
Total Fat 10.6g	14%
Saturated Fat 1.5g	8%
Cholesterol 0mg	0%
Sodium 112mg	5%
Total Carbohydrate 40.5g	15%
Dietary Fiber 4.1g	15%
Total Sugars 2.3g	
Protein 8.5g	
Vitamin D 0mcg	0%
Calcium 164mg	13%
Iron 2mg	13%
Potassium 75mg	2%

GINGER STICKY PORK

Are you looking for a satisfying, easy to cook a meal with pork? Ginger Sticky Pork is a great candidate for you and your family members with Ulcerative Colitis.

- Prep Time: 15 minutes
- Cook Time: 10 minutes
- Total Time: 25 minutes
- Serving: 6

Ingredients

- 1½ lb boneless, fat-removed pork tenderloin, cut into strips with ½ inch (~1.3cm) thickness
- 1 tablespoon extra virgin olive oil
- ½ cup honey or maple syrup

182

- 2 inches (~5cm) fresh ginger knob
- 1 tablespoon lemon juice
- 1 teaspoon salt
- ½ teaspoon black pepper
- 1 tablespoon garlic powder (optional)
- 1 tablespoon grape vinegar (optional)

Instructions

1. Heat extra virgin olive oil in a skillet over medium-high heat until shimmering.
2. Add your pork, salt, and pepper to the skillet. Brown one side first and then brown the other side of pork. Take out your pork.
3. Add ginger, lemon juice, grape vinegar (optional), garlic powder (optional), and honey to the pan. Stir and bring to boil.
4. When the sauce gets thick and sticky like honey, bring back your pork. Enjoy!

Cooking Tips:

- This dish can be served perfectly with white steamed rice.
- If the sauce gets very thick, add grape vinegar or sour grape juice or water.

UC-related Tips:

- Boil pork in water if you are in a severe flare-up. Then, take the pork out of boiling water and add them to your sticky sauce.
- If you cannot use honey, you can use maple syrup, ½ teaspoon of stevia or agave syrup.

- Do not use black pepper in your meal if you are in a severe flare-up.

Nutrition Facts

Servings: 6

Amount per serving

Calories 275

	% Daily Value*
Total Fat 6.4g	8%
Saturated Fat 1.7g	9%
Cholesterol 63mg	28%
Sodium 454mg	20%
Total Carbohydrate 24.9g	9%
Dietary Fiber 0.4g	1%
Total Sugars 23.5g	
Protein 30g	
Vitamin D 0mcg	0%
Calcium 12mg	1%
Iron 2mg	9%
Potassium 521mg	11%

GERMAN PORK SCHNITZEL

If you are looking for tender pork with a crispy crust, try German Pork Schnitzel. It is very easy to make it, and it is well-matched with baby carrots and potato garnishes.

- Prep Time: 20 minutes
- Cook Time: 15 minutes
- Total Time: 35 minutes
- Serving: 4

Ingredients

- 2 lbs boneless fatless pork tenderloins flattened into ½ inch (1.3cm) thick
- 3 large organic free-range eggs
- 2 cups bread crumbs or gluten-free bread crumbs
- ⅓ cup all-purpose flour or gluten-free flour
- 2 tablespoons extra virgin olive oil
- Lemon wedges for taste
- ½ teaspoon salt

- ½ teaspoon black pepper

Instructions

1. Pound your pork pieces with a mallet until it gets ½ inch thick.
2. In a medium bowl, mix flour, and pepper.
3. In another bowl, whisk three eggs.
4. In another bowl or plate, spread your breadcrumbs.
5. First, put both sides of pork cutlets in flour. Then, dip them in egg and then drip them into breadcrumbs using a fork.
6. Now, heat a large pan with extra virgin olive oil over medium heat. When the oil gets very hot, cook your cutlets for 5 minutes, each side until each side gets golden brown.
7. Enjoy the meal with lemon wedges!

Cooking Tips:

- This dish can be served perfectly with mashed potatoes. If you are lactose-intolerant, use lactose-free milk to make mashed potatoes.
- Use gluten-free bread crumbs and flour if you are gluten intolerant.

UC-related Tips:

- Do not use black pepper in your meal if you are in a severe flare-up.
- Use only one egg if you cannot tolerate eggs well during a flare-up.

Nutrition Facts

Servings: 4

Amount per serving

Calories **600**

	% Daily Value*
Total Fat 19.3g	25%
Saturated Fat 4.7g	23%
Cholesterol 243mg	81%
Sodium 979mg	43%
Total Carbohydrate 49.6g	18%
Dietary Fiber 2.9g	10%
Total Sugars 5.7g	
Protein 54.5g	
Vitamin D 12mcg	56%
Calcium 120mg	9%
Iron 6mg	33%
Potassium 169mg	4%

PINEAPPLE PORK

A delicious pork-based recipe that has been modified for Ulcerative Colitis patients.

- Prep Time: 5 minutes
- Cook Time: 25 minutes
- Total Time: 30 minutes
- Serving: 4

Ingredients

- 2 lbs skinless, boneless pork tenderloin
- 1 cup small pineapple, cut into small cubes
- 1 tablespoon peeled and grated ginger (~1 inch or ~2.5 cm)
- 2 tablespoons soy sauce
- 2 tablespoons balsamic vinegar
- 2 tablespoons extra virgin olive oil
- Salt and black pepper to taste
- 1 teaspoon garlic powder (optional)

Instructions

1. Mix ginger, garlic powder (optional), balsamic vinegar, and soy sauce in a small bowl.
2. Add salt and pepper to your pork.
3. Use a large skillet and cook both sides of your pork in it over medium heat with high-quality extra virgin olive oil until golden brown.
4. Check by a knife to see if the inside pork cooked or not. Remove the pork pieces from the skillet. Add your sauce to the pan and let it cooked for three more minutes.
5. Cook your pineapple in the same skillet for three minutes. If the sauce gets dry, add a little bit of water.
6. Bring back pork pieces to the skillet and let it cook for one more minute.

Cooking Tips:

- This dish can be served with steamed white rice.
- You can use peeled and poached peach cubes instead of pineapple.

UC-related Tips:

- Do not use black pepper or garlic powder if you are experiencing a severe flare-up.
- Vinegar may reduce inflammation in the colon. However, its sourness can annoy your gut. Try to use less vinegar if you are in a flare-up.

Nutrition Facts

Servings: 4

Amount per serving

Calories 375

	% Daily Value*
Total Fat 15.2g	19%
Saturated Fat 4g	20%
Cholesterol 132mg	44%
Sodium 533mg	23%
Total Carbohydrate 7.4g	3%
Dietary Fiber 0.7g	2%
Total Sugars 5.5g	
Protein 51.3g	
Vitamin D 0mcg	0%
Calcium 7mg	1%
Iron 2mg	10%
Potassium 68mg	1%

BALSAMIC-PEACH PORK

Balsamic-Peach Pork is a great and easy-to-cook meal with few ingredients. A fantastic combination of peach and honey gives the dish a lovely sweet taste.

- Prep Time: 10 minutes
- Cook Time: 20 minutes
- Total Time: 30 minutes
- Serving: 4

<u>Ingredients</u>

- 2 boneless pork tenderloins
- 2 sliced peeled peaches
- 6 oz low-fat feta cheese or lactose-free Swiss cheese
- ½ cup balsamic vinegar
- 1 tablespoon honey or maple syrup
- 2 tablespoons extra virgin olive oil
- 1 tablespoon fresh chopped oregano or thyme leaves
- Salt and black pepper to taste
- ½ cup fresh basil (optional)

<u>Instructions</u>

1. Mix cheese, balsamic vinegar, honey (or maple syrup), oregano, or thyme leaves in a bowl.
2. Add salt and pepper to your pork.
3. Use a large skillet and cook both sides of your pork in it over medium heat with high-quality extra virgin olive oil until golden brown.
4. Check by knife if inside pork cooked well. Remove the pork pieces from the skillet. Add your sauce to the pan and let it cooked for three more minutes.
5. Cook your peeled-off peaches in the same skillet for five minutes. If your sauce gets dry, add water a little bit.
6. Bring back pork pieces to the skillet and let it cook for two more minutes.
7. Garnish with fresh basil if you want. Enjoy!

Cooking Tips:

- This dish can be served well with steamed white rice.
- You can have lactose-free Havarti cheese instead of low-fat feta or Swiss cheese.

UC-related Tips:

- Do not use black pepper or many green basils if you are experiencing a severe flare-up.
- Vinegar can reduce inflammation in the colon. However, its sourness can annoy your gut. Try to use less vinegar if you are in a flare-up.
- If you cannot tolerate honey, remove honey from your recipe or use one tablespoon of stevia instead.

Nutrition Facts

Servings: 4

Amount per serving

Calories   **266**

	% Daily Value*
Total Fat 15.6g	20%
Saturated Fat 1.5g	8%
Cholesterol 31mg	10%
Sodium 476mg	21%
Total Carbohydrate 14.6g	5%
Dietary Fiber 1.7g	6%
Total Sugars 11.5g	
Protein 18.7g	
Vitamin D 1mcg	6%
Calcium 585mg	45%
Iron 2mg	11%
Potassium 365mg	8%

HONEY-TURMERIC PORK

If you are looking for a healthy dish, you are reading the right recipe. A short cooking-time Honey-Turmeric Pork is an excellent choice for Ulcerative Colitis patients who wants to have a rich pork-based main course.

- Prep Time: 15 minutes
- Cook Time: 15 minutes
- Total Time: 30 minutes
- Serving: 4

Ingredients

- 1¼ pounds chopped boneless, fat-removed pork tenderloin
- ½ cup plain yogurt or plain lactose-free yogurt
- ¼ cup honey or maple syrup
- 2 tablespoons extra virgin olive oil
- 3 small carrots
- 1½ teaspoons turmeric powder
- 3 tablespoons fresh lemon juice
- Salt and black pepper to taste
- 1 teaspoon garlic powder (optional)

- 3 small beets, sliced thin (optional)

Instructions

1. Mix plain yogurt, honey (or maple syrup), garlic powder (optional), turmeric, and lemon juice in a bowl.
2. Pour salt and pepper on your pork.
3. Use a large skillet and cook both sides of your pork in it over medium heat with high-quality extra virgin olive oil until golden brown.
4. Check by knife if inside pork cooked well. Remove the pork pieces from the skillet. Add your sauce to the pan and let it cooked for three more minutes.
5. Cook your peeled-off beets (optional) and carrots in a small skillet for 10 minutes as sides.
6. Bring back pork pieces to the skillet and let it cook for two more minutes. Enjoy it with carrot and beet sides!

Cooking Tips:

- This dish can be served well with steamed white rice or noodles.
- If you are lactose-intolerant, use lactose-free plain yogurt or remove yogurt from the recipe.

UC-related Tips:

- Do not use black pepper or beets if you are experiencing a severe flare-up.
- If you cannot tolerate honey, remove honey from your recipe or use one tablespoon of stevia instead.

Nutrition Facts

Servings: 4

Amount per serving

Calories   **624**

	% Daily Value*
Total Fat 18.7g	24%
Saturated Fat 6.2g	26%
Cholesterol 229mg	76%
Sodium 235mg	10%
Total Carbohydrate 26.4g	10%
Dietary Fiber 1.9g	7%
Total Sugars 22.2g	
Protein 84.1g	
Vitamin D 0mcg	0%
Calcium 98mg	8%
Iron 5mg	28%
Potassium 1633mg	35%

GRILLED LEAN BEEF KEBAB

Ulcerative Colitis patients have to significantly reduce red meat in their diet as typically, red meat meals are harder to digest, and they can cause flare-ups. Extra-lean beef with no fats is recommended for Ulcerative Colitis patients who want to consume red meats. Another fabulous alternative to red meat is Ostrich meat. It tastes very similar to lean beef, but it has less fat, cholesterol. It is high in calcium, iron, and protein. It is highly recommended for Ulcerative Colitis patients to include Ostrich beef in their diet once a week.

- Prep Time: 10 minutes
- Marinate Time: 60 minutes
- Cook Time: 20 minutes
- Total Time: 90 minutes
- Serving: 4

Ingredients

- 2 lbs extra lean beef or lamb meat
- ½ cup plain yogurt or plain lactose-free yogurt
- 1 small kiwi
- 1 onion (thinly sliced)

- 1 tablespoon extra virgin olive oil
- 4 tablespoons fresh lemon juice
- Salt and black pepper to taste

Instructions

1. Cut extra lean beef/lamb into small 1-inch (~2.54cm) cubes.
2. Ina large bowl, marinate your beef/lamb with plain yogurt, onion, kiwi, lemon juice, olive oil, salt, and pepper.
3. Cover the top bowl, fridge it and Let it marinate for 1 hour.
4. Skewer your kebab cubes or just grill both sides like a steak. Ten minutes grill would suffice for medium kebabs, and 20 minutes grill would suffice for well-done kebabs.

Cooking Tips:

- You do not necessarily need to cut your beef/lamb into cubes. You can flatten them by mallet and make a fantastic steak.
- Kiwi melts your kebab and makes it very juicy.
- This dish can be served well with steamed white rice.
- If you are lactose-intolerant, use lactose-free plain yogurt or remove yogurt from the recipe.

UC-related Tips:

- Do not use black pepper or onion if you are experiencing a severe flare-up.

Nutrition Facts	
Servings: 4	
Amount per serving	
Calories	**499**
	% Daily Value*
Total Fat 18.3g	23%
Saturated Fat 6.3g	31%
Cholesterol 205mg	68%
Sodium 176mg	8%
Total Carbohydrate 7.9g	3%
Dietary Fiber 1.2g	4%
Total Sugars 5.4g	
Protein 71.2g	
Vitamin D 0mcg	0%
Calcium 73mg	6%
Iron 43mg	238%
Potassium 1104mg	23%

HUNGARIAN GOULASH

Goulash is a great traditional stew full of healthy ingredients. Ulcerative Colitis patients need to add more bone, beef, chicken, or vegetable broth meals in their diet. Hungarian Goulash is a great option that can be added to your weekly meal plan.

- Prep Time: 30 minutes
- Cook Time: 90 minutes
- Total Time: 120 minutes
- Serving: 6

<u>Ingredients</u>

- 1½ lbs extra lean beef trimmed into 1 inch (~2.54 cm) cubes
- 2 cups bone/beef broth or tap water
- 2 tablespoons extra virgin olive oil
- 2 tablespoons lemon juice
- ½ tablespoon turmeric
- 1 teaspoon salt
- ¼ teaspoon pepper
- 1 cup carrots

- 2 cups potatoes, cut into 1 inch (~2.54cm) cubes
- 1 tablespoon tomato paste (optional)

Instructions

1. One a large pan or a pot, heat olive oil, turmeric, tomato paste (optional), and pepper over medium heat.
2. Add your extra lean beef and stir for 5 minutes.
3. Add water or bone/beef broth slowly to your pot. Then, cover and let it cook for 50 minutes over low heat until tender.
4. Add potatoes and let it cook for 20 more minutes. Add salt and lemon juice. Then, add the carrots and cook the stew for 15 more minutes. Enjoy!

Cooking Tips:

- This dish can be served well with steamed white rice.
- Anytime the stew gets very thick, add more water into it.

UC-related Tips:

- Do not use black pepper or tomato paste if you are experiencing a severe flare-up.

Nutrition Facts

Servings: 6

Amount per serving

Calories 309

	% Daily Value*
Total Fat 12.4g	16%
Saturated Fat 3.5g	18%
Cholesterol 101mg	34%
Sodium 734mg	32%
Total Carbohydrate 10.5g	4%
Dietary Fiber 1.8g	8%
Total Sugars 1.8g	
Protein 37.1g	
Vitamin D 0mcg	0%
Calcium 17mg	1%
Iron 22mg	123%
Potassium 810mg	17%

TOMATO FREE SPAGHETTI BOLOGNESE

Many of Ulcerative Colitis patients cannot well-tolerated tomatoes and tomato pastes, which can negatively affect their regular cooking habits using tomatoes inside meals. Let us try a great Spaghetti Bolognese tomato-free! Yes, you read correctly! Enjoy a tomato-free Italian dish now!

- Prep Time: 15 minutes
- Cook Time: 25 minutes
- Total Time: 40 minutes
- Serving: 4

<u>Ingredients</u>

- 1 lb (~500 s) extra lean ground beef
- 0.65 lb (~300 g) spaghetti or gluten-free spaghetti
- 1 cup organic unsalted chicken stock
- 1 tablespoon extra virgin olive oil
- 1 tablespoon soy sauce
- 2 tablespoons maple syrup
- 1 teaspoon dried oregano or oregano powder
- ½ teaspoon dried thyme
- 1 teaspoon dried basil

- ½ tablespoon turmeric
- 1 teaspoon salt
- ¼ teaspoon pepper
- 1 tablespoon of Parmesan or any lactose-free cheese (optional)

Instructions

1. Golden both sides of your extra lean ground beef in a large pan with extra virgin olive oil over high heat.
2. Add soy sauce, honey (or maple syrup), salt, pepper, turmeric, and chicken stock to your ground beef. Let it thicken and have it cooked for one more minute.
3. At the same time, prepare your spaghetti according to its package recipe with a pinch of salt and a little bit of olive oil.
4. Take your spaghetti out of boiling water and put it in your sauce.
5. Season it with dried basil.

Cooking Tips:

- You can add some lactose-free cheese to this recipe if you are lactose intolerant.
- If your sauce thickened more than desired, add some tap water or spaghetti boiling water.

UC-related Tips:

- Do not use black pepper, Parmesan, or fresh herbs if you are experiencing a severe flare-up.

Nutrition Facts	
Servings: 4	

Amount per serving	
Calories	**475**

	% Daily Value*
Total Fat 12.9g	17%
Saturated Fat 4.2g	21%
Cholesterol 141mg	47%
Sodium 1092mg	47%
Total Carbohydrate 49.1g	18%
Dietary Fiber 0.5g	2%
Total Sugars 6.3g	
Protein 38.8g	
Vitamin D 0mcg	0%
Calcium 42mg	3%
Iron 7mg	37%
Potassium 593mg	13%

LAMB/BEEF LIVER STEW

A great stew with excellent sources of Iron, Vitamin A, D, and B12 for Ulcerative Colitis patients. However, the lamb/beef liver has to be used with caution in patients who have high cholesterol.

- Prep Time: 10 minutes
- Cook Time: 20 minutes
- Total Time: 30 minutes
- Serving: 4

Ingredients

- 1 lb (~500 g) lamb/beef liver, cut in 1 inch (~2.54cm) cubes
- 1 cup of organic unsalted bone/beef broth
- 2 tablespoons extra virgin olive oil
- 2 teaspoons turmeric
- 1 teaspoon salt
- ½ teaspoon pepper
- 1 potato, cut into 1 inch (~2.54cm) cubes (optional)
- 2 tablespoons tomato paste (optional)

Instructions

1. Fully cook your lamb/beef liver in a large pan with extra virgin olive oil, turmeric, salt and pepper, potatoes (optional), and tomato paste (optional) over medium heat for 15 minutes.
2. Add your bone/beef broth to your livers. Cook for 5 minutes until thickened.

Cooking Tips:

- You can add 1 tablespoon of flour or gluten-free flour if your stew is not getting thick.
- If your stew thickened more than desired, add some hot water to it.

UC-related Tips:

- Do not use black pepper and tomato paste if you are experiencing a flare-up.
- If you are in high cholesterol, you can substitute the liver with the extra lean ostrich.

Nutrition Facts
Servings: 4

Amount per serving

Calories   **273**

% Daily Value*

Total Fat 12.8g	16%
Saturated Fat 2.8g	14%
Cholesterol 432mg	144%
Sodium 860mg	37%
Total Carbohydrate 7g	3%
Dietary Fiber 0.3g	1%
Total Sugars 0.2g	
Protein 31.4g	
Vitamin D 0mcg	0%
Calcium 13mg	1%
Iron 8mg	43%
Potassium 481mg	10%

GRILLED HONEY SALMON

Try a yummy grilled honey salmon dish. Those who are in a severe flare-up, can your maple syrup in moderation instead of honey.

- Prep Time: 5 minutes
- Cook Time: 25 minutes
- Total Time: 30 minutes
- Serving: 4

Ingredients:

- 2 lbs (~1 kg) salmon fillets
- ¼ cup honey or maple syrup
- 1 tablespoon extra virgin olive oil
- 1 teaspoon turmeric powder
- 1 tablespoon fresh thyme leaves
- Salt and black pepper, to taste
- 1 teaspoon garlic powder (optional)

Directions:

1. Choose a medium bowl and whisk honey (or maple syrup), turmeric, thyme leaves, garlic (optional), extra virgin olive oil, salt, and pepper together.
2. Preheat your oven to 375 °F.
3. Pour your sauce over the salmon.
4. Put your salmon in the oven and let it cook for 20 minutes (until inside cooks well).
5. Enjoy!

Cooking Tips:

- If your salmon is thicker, you have to increase the cooking time until inside cooks well.
- You can add balsamic vinegar or sour grape juice to your sauce if you can tolerate it.

- You can cover your salmon with foil for having a juicy texture.

<u>UC-related Tips:</u>

- Do not use black pepper in your meal if you are experiencing a flare-up.
- If you cannot tolerate honey, try maple syrup, agave syrup or a teaspoon of stevia.

Nutrition Facts

Servings: 4

Amount per serving

Calories	398
	% Daily Value*
Total Fat 17.6g	23%
Saturated Fat 2.5g	13%
Cholesterol 100mg	33%
Sodium 101mg	4%
Total Carbohydrate 18.3g	7%
Dietary Fiber 0.4g	2%
Total Sugars 17.4g	
Protein 44.2g	
Vitamin D 0mcg	0%
Calcium 95mg	7%
Iron 3mg	15%
Potassium 902mg	19%

OVEN-BASED SALMON AND POTATO

A great mix of salmon and oven-baked potatoes give you a joyful lunch or dinner meal!

- Prep Time: 5 minutes
- Cook Time: 25 minutes
- Total Time: 30 minutes
- Serving: 4

<u>Ingredients</u>

- 4 salmon filets, about 6 ounces each
- 2 medium potatoes, sliced into very thin chips
- 3 tablespoons extra-virgin olive oil, divided

- 2 oranges
- 2 lemons
- Salt and pepper to taste

Instructions

1. Choose a small bowl and whisk orange juice, lemon juice, 1 tablespoon of extra virgin olive oil, salt, and pepper all together to have a juicy sauce.
2. Marinate your salmon with the sauce.
3. Slice potatoes very thin. Drizzle potatoes with two tablespoons of extra virgin olive oil and a pinch of salt.
4. Preheat your oven to 375 °F.
5. Choose a long foil sheet, put potatoes first, and fill the top with your salmon. Close your foil and let the salmon cook for about 25 minutes until inside cooks well.
6. Enjoy!

Cooking Tips:

- If your salmon is very thick, you have to increase the cooking time until inside cooks well.
- Check both salmon and your potato to be cooked. If required, return your salmon and potato to the over for five more minutes until perfection.

UC-related Tips:

- Do not use black pepper in your meal if you are experiencing a flare-up.
- If you cannot tolerate orange juice, remove it from the recipe.

Nutrition Facts

Servings: 4

Amount per serving

Calories **443**

	% Daily Value*
Total Fat 21.8g	28%
Saturated Fat 3.1g	16%
Cholesterol 76mg	26%
Sodium 84mg	4%
Total Carbohydrate 28.4g	10%
Dietary Fiber 4.9g	18%
Total Sugars 10g	
Protein 37.4g	
Vitamin D 0mcg	0%
Calcium 117mg	9%
Iron 2mg	11%
Potassium 1248mg	27%

LEMON STEAMED HALIBUT WITH WHITE RICE

A great dish with healthy ingredients for Ulcerative Colitis patients. You can substitute halibut with any other fishes you would like to have.

- Prep Time: 10 minutes
- Cook Time: 30 minutes
- Total Time: 40 minutes
- Serving: 6

Ingredients

- 6 skinless and boneless halibut fillets, about 6 ounces each
- 2 cups steamed white rice
- 1 tablespoon extra virgin olive oil
- 1 lemon, sliced very thin
- 4 tablespoons lemon juice
- 1 teaspoon ginger powder
- Salt and pepper to taste
- Lemon wedges to garnish
- 1 teaspoon garlic powder (optional)

Instructions

1. Choose a small bowl and whisk lemon juice, ginger powder, garlic powder (optional), extra virgin olive oil, salt, and pepper all together to have a juicy sauce.
2. Marinate your halibut with the sauce.
3. Preheat your oven to 375 °F.
4. Choose a long foil sheet, put halibut in your foil sheet, and close it. Let it cook for about 25 minutes until inside cooks well.
5. Open the foil sheet, put thin lemon slices on top of your halibut for 5 minutes, and close the foil sheet again.
6. Steam your white rice. Open your foil sheet and put halibut on top of the rice.
7. Garnish with lemon wedges. Enjoy!

Cooking Tips:

- If your halibut is very thick, you have to increase the cooking time until inside cooks well.

UC-related Tips:

- Do not use black pepper in your meal if you are experiencing a flare-up.
- Do not use garlic powder if you cannot tolerate it.

Nutrition Facts

Servings: 6

Amount per serving

Calories   **568**

	% Daily Value*
Total Fat 9.5g	12%
Saturated Fat 1.4g	7%
Cholesterol 93mg	31%
Sodium 161mg	7%
Total Carbohydrate 50.2g	18%
Dietary Fiber 1.3g	4%
Total Sugars 0.3g	
Protein 65g	
Vitamin D 0mcg	0%
Calcium 33mg	3%
Iron 18mg	67%
Potassium 1396mg	30%

THUNFISCH PIZZA

Thunfisch Pizza is an excellent German-based pizza with Tuna. The classic recipe has been modified to be tolerated by most Ulcerative Colitis patients.

- Prep Time: 5 minutes
- Cook Time: 15 minutes
- Total Time: 20 minutes
- Serving: 4

Ingredients

- 2 medium-size gluten-free pizza crusts
- 1 cup shredded mozzarella or lactose-free cheese pizza
- Two 6.5 oz tuna can on oil or water
- 2 tablespoons organic mayonnaise
- 2 teaspoons dried ground oregano
- Salt to taste

Instructions

1. Place your gluten-free pizza crusts on a non-stick pizza pan or bake sheet.

2. Spread your organic mayo on your crust.
3. Gently put tuna on your pizza crust.
4. Sprinkle with mozzarella or lactose-free cheese
5. Let it bake at 400 °F for 10 minutes. Then, broil on the same heat for five more minutes until cheese melted.

Cooking Tips:

- You can use any other white sauces such as a béchamel sauce (explained before in Fettuccine Alfredo recipe) instead of mayonnaise.

UC-related Tips:

- If you are lactose intolerant, use lactose-free or dairy-free cheese pizza.
- Use mayonnaise only if you can tolerate it. If you cannot tolerate, you can make a béchamel sauce (explain before in Fettuccine Alfredo recipe) instead.

Nutrition Facts

Servings: 4

Amount per serving	
Calories	**297**
	% Daily Value*
Total Fat 13g	17%
Saturated Fat 2.8g	14%
Cholesterol 33mg	11%
Sodium 333mg	14%
Total Carbohydrate 17g	6%
Dietary Fiber 0.8g	3%
Total Sugars 1.5g	
Protein 26.8g	
Vitamin D 0mcg	0%
Calcium 21mg	2%
Iron 1mg	5%
Potassium 310mg	7%

AVOCADO TUNA PITA

A very fast sandwich you can prepare at home for your lunch or dinner. You can even have a smaller portion of avocado tuna as a breakfast or as a snack at work.

- Prep Time: 10 minutes
- Cook Time: 0 minutes
- Total Time: 10 minutes
- Serving: 4

Ingredients

- 2 avocados
- 2 tablespoons organic mayonnaise
- 1 teaspoon cumin powder
- 1 can of tuna in olive oil or water
- ¼ cup apple, chopped and peeled off
- 4 Pita bread or any gluten-free bread
- 1 teaspoon Dijon mustard (optional)
- Salt to taste
- Pepper to taste (optional)

Instructions

1. Choose a small bowl. Mix tuna with smashed avocado with mayo, cumin powder, peeled off apple (cut into small pieces), mustard (optional), salt, and pepper (optional).
2. Open each of your pita bread from the corner and spoon the mix inside.
3. Roll the pita. Enjoy!

Cooking Tips:

- You can make this sandwich without mayonnaise sauce, as well.

UC-related Tips:

- Do not use black pepper, cumin powder, or mustard if you are experiencing a flare-up.

Nutrition Facts

Servings: 4

Amount per serving

Calories   **491**

	% Daily Value*
Total Fat 26.5g	34%
Saturated Fat 5.3g	27%
Cholesterol 16mg	5%
Sodium 442mg	19%
Total Carbohydrate 46g	17%
Dietary Fiber 8.5g	30%
Total Sugars 3.2g	
Protein 19.4g	
Vitamin D 0mcg	0%
Calcium 71mg	5%
Iron 5mg	16%
Potassium 733mg	16%

TROUT WITH ORANGE

Great classic seafood that typically serves with steamed white rice. It is recommended to make this dish with bitter or blood oranges.

- Prep Time: 20 minutes
- Cook Time: 30 minutes
- Total Time: 50 minutes
- Serving: 6

Ingredients

- Large fresh trout, 1.5 lbs each
- 3 oranges
- 1 tablespoon lemon juice
- 1 tablespoon extra virgin olive oil
- ½ teaspoon turmeric powder
- Salt & pepper to taste
- 1 teaspoon garlic powder (optional)

Instructions

1. Choose a medium bowl and whisk lemon juice, orange juice, turmeric powder, garlic powder

(optional), extra virgin olive oil, salt, and pepper all together to have a juicy sauce.
2. Marinate your trout with the sauce. For better taste, you may need to let it rest at room temperature for 30 minutes.
3. Preheat your oven to 375 °F.
4. Choose a long foil sheet, put trout in your foil sheet and close it. Let it cook for about 25 minutes until inside cooks well.
5. Enjoy!

Cooking Tips:

- Check your trout until inside cooked well. You may need more minutes for perfection.
- This dish can be served with potatoes or steamed white rice.
- You can substitute orange with mango or lemon juice if you like to try other great flavors.

UC-related Tips:

- Do not use black pepper and garlic powder if you are experiencing a flare-up.

Nutrition Facts
Servings: 4

Amount per serving

Calories	391
	% Daily Value*
Total Fat 16.9g	22%
Saturated Fat 2.8g	14%
Cholesterol 115mg	38%
Sodium 105mg	5%
Total Carbohydrate 16.5g	6%
Dietary Fiber 3.4g	12%
Total Sugars 13g	
Protein 42.8g	
Vitamin D 0mcg	0%
Calcium 141mg	11%
Iron 3mg	18%
Potassium 960mg	21%

CHICKEN AND SHRIMP TERIYAKI

A lovely Edo-style mix of chicken and shrimp with healthy ingredients for Ulcerative Colitis patients.

- Prep Time: 5 minutes
- Cook Time: 20 minutes
- Total Time: 25 minutes
- Serving: 4

Ingredients

- 2 lbs (~1 kg) organic chicken breast, chopped in cubes
- 24 shrimps, peeled and deveined
- 1 tablespoon ginger powder, divided
- 2 tablespoons extra virgin olive oil
- ½ teaspoon turmeric
- ⅓ cup gluten-free and sodium-reduced soy sauce
- ⅓ cup of cold water
- 3 teaspoons arrowroot powder
- ¼ cup honey, or maple syrup
- Salt & pepper to taste

Instructions

1. In a medium bowl, whisk ginger powder, one tablespoon of olive oil, soy sauce, arrowroot powder, honey (or maple syrup), water, salt, and pepper to make a juicy teriyaki sauce.
2. Let Teriyaki sauce rest in the fridge for 5 minutes.
3. In a large pan, add one tablespoon of olive oil and cook chicken over medium heat until golden brown both sides.

4. Add your sauce and shrimp to the pan. Stir and mix for 5 minutes until thickened.
5. Enjoy!

Cooking Tips:

- You can serve this dish with steamed white rice or rice noodles.

UC-related Tips:

- Do not use black pepper if you are experiencing a severe flare-up.
- Use maple syrup or stevia (1 teaspoon) if you cannot tolerate honey.

Nutrition Facts
Servings: 4

Amount per serving
Calories   **553**

	% Daily Value*
Total Fat 15.1g	19%
Saturated Fat 1.7g	9%
Cholesterol 423mg	141%
Sodium 1639mg	71%
Total Carbohydrate 20g	7%
Dietary Fiber 0.4g	1%
Total Sugars 12.1g	
Protein 79.6g	
Vitamin D 0mcg	1%
Calcium 151mg	12%
Iron 2mg	12%
Potassium 1175mg	25%

LEMON SHRIMP WITH WHITE RICE

Lemon Shrimp with steamed white rice is very easy to make and a healthy dish you can have in your weekly diet.

- Prep Time: 5 minutes
- Cook Time: 20 minutes
- Total Time: 25 minutes
- Serving: 4

Ingredients

- 24 shrimps, peeled and deveined
- 2 tablespoons extra virgin olive oil, divided
- ½ teaspoon turmeric powder
- 4 tablespoons lemon juice
- 3 cups of white rice
- 1 teaspoon salt & pepper
- 1 teaspoon garlic powder (optional)

Instructions

1. In a small bowl, whisk lemon juice, garlic powder (optional), one tablespoon of olive oil, turmeric powder, salt, and pepper to make a sauce.
2. Cook your rice according to its package instructions.
3. Add one tablespoon of high-quality extra virgin olive oil in a pan and cook shrimp over medium heat for 5-7 minutes.
4. Add your sauce into the pan. Stir and mix well for 5 minutes.
5. Enjoy!

Cooking Tips:

- You can serve the lemon shrimp with rice noodles instead of white rice.

UC-related Tips:

- Do not use black pepper and garlic powder if you are experiencing a severe flare-up.

Nutrition Facts

Servings: 4

Amount per serving

Calories 729

	% Daily Value*
Total Fat 10.3g	13%
Saturated Fat 2.1g	10%
Cholesterol 278mg	93%
Sodium 332mg	14%
Total Carbohydrate 113.8g	41%
Dietary Fiber 2.1g	7%
Total Sugars 0.5g	
Protein 40.2g	
Vitamin D 0mcg	0%
Calcium 162mg	12%
Iron 7mg	37%
Potassium 416mg	9%

HONEY PRAWN LINGUINE

Are you looking for an Italian seafood linguine recipe for Ulcerative Colitis patients? You have to try this delicious main course.

- Prep Time: 5 minutes
- Cook Time: 20 minutes
- Total Time: 25 minutes
- Serving: 4

Ingredients:

- 1 lb (~500 gr) prawns, peeled and deveined
- 1 lb (~500 gr) cooked linguine or any gluten-free pasta
- 2 tablespoons extra virgin olive oil, divided
- 4 tablespoons honey or maple syrup
- ½ cup carrot
- ½ cup of water
- Salt and black pepper to taste
- ¼ cup green onion (only if tolerated)
- 1 teaspoon garlic powder (optional)

Instructions

1. Whisk honey (or maple syrup), garlic powder (optional), one tablespoon of olive oil, carrot, green onion, pepper, and salt in a proper bowl to make a sauce.
2. Cook your linguini according to its package instructions.
3. Add one tablespoon of high-quality extra virgin olive oil in a medium-size pan and cook prawns over medium heat for 5-7 minutes.
4. Add your sauce into the pan. Stir and mix well for 5 minutes until sauce gets thick.
5. Add pasta to your sauce and mix all well. Enjoy!

Cooking Tips:

- You can serve honey prawn linguine with rice noodles or any other kinds of pasta instead of linguini.

UC-related Tips:

- Do not use black pepper, green onion, and garlic powder if you are experiencing a severe flare-up.
- You can use maple syrup, agave syrup, or a teaspoon of stevia if you cannot tolerate honey.

Nutrition Facts

Servings: 4

Amount per serving

Calories 592

	% Daily Value*
Total Fat 11.5g	15%
Saturated Fat 2g	10%
Cholesterol 322mg	107%
Sodium 317mg	14%
Total Carbohydrate 82.7g	30%
Dietary Fiber 0.5g	2%
Total Sugars 18g	
Protein 38.9g	
Vitamin D 0mcg	0%
Calcium 128mg	10%
Iron 4mg	24%
Potassium 461mg	10%

DESSERTS

PINEAPPLE CAKE SUNDAES

A delicious dessert with pineapple, cinnamon, and ice cream. Substantially modified to be consumed by Ulcerative Colitis patients.

- Prep Time: 15 minutes
- Total Time: 15 minutes
- Serving: 4

Ingredients

- 2 tablespoons extra virgin olive oil
- ¼ cup brown sugar or one tablespoon honey
- 1 cup pineapple, chopped
- 1-pint lactose-free vanilla ice cream or sorbet
- 1½ cup vanilla loaf pound cake
- 1 tablespoon maple syrup
- ¼ teaspoon cinnamon powder

Instructions

- In a medium skillet, heat extra virgin olive oil over medium heat. Add brown sugar, cinnamon, and honey. Stir well until brown with a soft texture.
- Add pineapple and let it cook for two-three more minutes. Remove from heat.
- Preheat oven to 375 °F. Bake your cake for about 8-10 minutes until toasted.
- Crumble vanilla loaf pound cake and place it on top of ice cream scoops (or sorbets). Pour maple syrup on top.
- Add pineapple sauce. Serve and enjoy!

Cooking Tips:

- You can mix the pineapple sauce with any cold plain or vanilla yogurt instead of ice cream.

UC-related Tips:

- Always try to consume less sugar. Instead, you can use honey. If you cannot tolerate honey well, you can use maple syrup or stevia.

Nutrition Facts

Servings: 4

Amount per serving

Calories 213

	% Daily Value*
Total Fat 10.8g	14%
Saturated Fat 2.6g	13%
Cholesterol 12mg	4%
Sodium 54mg	2%
Total Carbohydrate 29g	11%
Dietary Fiber 0.7g	3%
Total Sugars 23.5g	
Protein 1.4g	
Vitamin D 0mcg	0%
Calcium 41mg	3%
Iron 1mg	3%
Potassium 78mg	2%

APPLE-GINGER SUNDAES

This summer sundae is based on a great combination of apple, ginger, and ice cream.

- Prep Time: 20 minutes
- Total Time: 20 minutes
- Serving: 4

Ingredients

- 2 apples, peeled and sliced
- 2 tablespoons extra virgin olive oil
- 2 tablespoons brown sugar or two tablespoon honey
- 6 tablespoons organic no added sugar, apple juice
- ½ teaspoon cornstarch
- 2 cup lactose-free vanilla ice cream or sorbet
- ¼ teaspoon freshly grated ginger

Instructions

- In a large skillet, heat extra virgin olive oil over medium heat. Add apple and ginger and cook for three minutes until tender. Add brown sugar or honey and stir well for 1-2 minutes.
- In a bowl, mix cornstarch and apple juice and pour the mix into the skillet. Cook all mix until thickened.
- Cool for 2-4 minutes.
- Scoop your ice cream or sorbet in a proper dessert plate. Pour your apple ginger mix on top.
- Serve and enjoy!

Cooking Tips:

- You can mix the apple ginger sauce with any cold plain or vanilla yogurt instead of ice cream.

UC-related Tips:

- Always try to consume less sugar. Instead, you can use honey. If you cannot tolerate honey well, you can use maple syrup or stevia.
- If you cannot tolerate cornstarch well, use all-purpose white flour or rice flour.

Nutrition Facts

Servings: 4

Amount per serving	
Calories	**212**

	% Daily Value*
Total Fat 10.7g	14%
Saturated Fat 3.3g	16%
Cholesterol 10mg	3%
Sodium 20mg	1%
Total Carbohydrate 29.7g	11%
Dietary Fiber 2.7g	10%
Total Sugars 25.2g	
Protein 1.3g	
Vitamin D 0mcg	0%
Calcium 46mg	4%
Iron 1mg	3%
Potassium 151mg	3%

BANANA LEMON TRIFLE

If you want to try a different delicious dessert, you have to make Banana Lemon Trifle.

- Prep Time: 10 minutes
- Total Time: 20 minutes
- Serving: 6

Ingredients

- 4 packs instant vanilla pudding or gluten-free vanilla pudding
- 3 packs shortbread cookies, or gluten-free shortbread cookies
- ½ cup low fat cow milk or almond milk
- 3 bananas, sliced
- 1 tablespoon lemon juice
- Lemon zest

- 4-5 fresh mint leaves

<u>Instructions</u>

- In a large bowl, prepare vanilla pudding according to package instructions. Then mix pudding with lemon juice, lemon zest, and almond milk.
- Top the bowl with shredded shortbread cookies and sliced banana. Garnish with mint leaves.

<u>Cooking Tips:</u>

- You can top the bowl with cinnamon powder as well.

<u>UC-related Tips:</u>

- Make sure you can tolerate mint leaves. Otherwise, do not use it.
- When in a flare-up, do not use milk. Instead, use boiling water.

Nutrition Facts

Servings: 6

Amount per serving

Calories	481
	% Daily Value*
Total Fat 11.2g	14%
Saturated Fat 6.4g	32%
Cholesterol 28mg	9%
Sodium 1033mg	45%
Total Carbohydrate 94.1g	34%
Dietary Fiber 2.6g	9%
Total Sugars 74.3g	
Protein 2.4g	
Vitamin D 0mcg	0%
Calcium 21mg	2%
Iron 1mg	4%
Potassium 253mg	5%

WARM APPLE CRUMBLE

Warm apple crumble is a quick dessert to make for yourself and your family.

- Prep Time: 15 minutes
- Cook Time: 15 minutes
- Total Time: 30 minutes
- Serving: 4

Ingredients

- 2.5 cups apple, peeled and sliced
- 1 teaspoon vanilla extract
- 2 tablespoons sugar or honey
- ¼ cup shredded coconut
- 1 teaspoon cinnamon powder, divided
- 2 tablespoons extra virgin olive oil
- Lactose-free vanilla ice cream or sorbet (optional)

Instructions

1. In a medium bowl, mix apple, with vanilla, sugar or honey, and half-teaspoon cinnamon powder.
2. Preheat oven to 350 °F.
3. Choose a proper baking dish. Place the mix in it.
4. Bake apples until slightly get golden (about 12-15 minutes).
5. Serve the apple crumble warm (with or without vanilla ice cream or sorbet). Garnish with shredded coconut. Enjoy!

Cooking Tips:

- Your cooking time highly depends on how thin you sliced apples. Keep your eyes on apples to avoid overcooking.

UC-related Tips:

- Always try to consume less sugar. Instead, you can use honey. If you cannot tolerate honey well, you can use maple syrup or stevia.
- When in a flare-up, do not have ice cream and shredded coconut with your apple crumble.

Nutrition Facts

Servings: 4

Amount per serving	
Calories	**177**
	% Daily Value*
Total Fat 8.9g	11%
Saturated Fat 2.5g	12%
Cholesterol 0mg	0%
Sodium 2mg	0%
Total Carbohydrate 28.6g	10%
Dietary Fiber 4.1g	15%
Total Sugars 21g	
Protein 0.6g	
Vitamin D 0mcg	0%
Calcium 7mg	1%
Iron 1mg	8%
Potassium 171mg	4%

GINGER FRUIT SHERBET

Try tasting new! A fantastic sherbet made from ginger, orange, and pineapple.

- Prep Time: 5 minutes
- Freeze Time: 20 minutes
- Total Time: 25 minutes
- Serving: 4

Ingredients

- 1 cup pineapple, diced
- 5 tablespoons orange marmalade/jam
- 2 cups orange, lemon, pineapple or lime sherbet
- 1 tablespoon freshly grated ginger
- ¼ teaspoon vanilla

Instructions

- In a large bowl, mix well all ingredients together.
- Chill the bowl for 15 minutes in your freezer.
- Remove from the freezer and refrigerate for five more minutes.
- Remove from the fridge. Stir the mix a bit, and enjoy it!

Making Tips:

- Add one more tablespoon of freshly grated ginger or ginger powder if you want to have a ginger flavor more.
- Try to find sugar-free marmalade or jam. If you cannot find it, you can make it fast at home by mixing orange, orange zest, and honey. Then, refrigerate it for an hour.

UC-related Tips:

- Orange can irritate the gut in some Ulcerative Colitis patients. Make sure you can tolerate orange. If you cannot, make a pineapple version by using a pineapple-honey mixture instead of orange marmalade.

Nutrition Facts

Servings: 4

Amount per serving	
Calories	**147**
	% Daily Value*
Total Fat 0.6g	1%
Saturated Fat 0.3g	1%
Cholesterol 3mg	1%
Sodium 23mg	1%
Total Carbohydrate 36.6g	13%
Dietary Fiber 0.9g	3%
Total Sugars 30.1g	
Protein 0.9g	
Vitamin D 0mcg	0%
Calcium 27mg	2%
Iron 0mg	2%
Potassium 73mg	2%

APPLE QUESADILLAS

If you can tolerate tortilla, then this dessert is an excellent option for you to make. It perfectly comes with ice cream on top.

- Prep Time: 10 minutes
- Cook Time: 10 minutes
- Total Time: 20 minutes
- Serving: 4-6

Ingredients

- 4 pieces of wheat tortillas
- 1 cup old cheddar cheese, shredded
- 1 tablespoon extra virgin olive oil
- 2 large apples, peeled, cored and skin removed
- 2 tablespoons brown sugar or honey
- 4 tablespoons lactose-free ice cream or sorbet

Instructions

1. Preheat oven to 375 °F.
2. Place your tortillas on a proper baking sheet. Sprinkle extra virgin olive oil, and top with cheddar, sugar or honey, and thinly sliced apples on half of each tortilla.
3. Wrap tortilla by folding the other half towards the half with mixture.
4. Bake quesadillas for about 7-10 minutes until golden.
5. Scoop ice cream or sorbet and top it with your apple mix. Enjoy!

Cooking Tips:

- You can use poached apple or warmed canned apple instead. Dice them and top with other ingredients. Cook for 5 minutes.

<u>UC-related Tips:</u>

- Always try to consume less sugar. Instead, you can use honey. If you cannot tolerate honey well, you can use maple syrup or stevia.
- When in a flare-up, do not have ice cream with your apple quesadillas.

Nutrition Facts

Servings: 6

Amount per serving	
Calories	**323**
	% Daily Value*
Total Fat 19.4g	25%
Saturated Fat 7.7g	38%
Cholesterol 35mg	12%
Sodium 155mg	7%
Total Carbohydrate 31.2g	11%
Dietary Fiber 7.1g	25%
Total Sugars 20g	
Protein 13.4g	
Vitamin D 0mcg	0%
Calcium 56mg	4%
Iron 0mg	2%
Potassium 84mg	2%

MIDDLE-EASTERN RICE PUDDING

Rice pudding is a well-known dessert everywhere. Try a luxurious taste of new rice pudding for Ulcerative Colitis patients!

- Prep Time: 10 minutes
- Cook Time: 30 minutes
- Total Time: 40 minutes
- Serving: 4-6

<u>Ingredients</u>

- 1 cup white rice
- 2 cups low fat milk or lactose-free milk
- ¾ cup sugar, honey or maple syrup
- ½ teaspoon grated cinnamon
- 2 tablespoons extra virgin olive oil
- 2 cups of water
- ½ cup rosewater (optional)

Instructions

1. In a medium pot, put rice and add boiling water. Let the rice boil over low heat until all water evaporates.
2. Add milk until boiled. Stir consistently.
3. Add sugar or honey and rose water (optional) and stir for 3-5 more minutes. Add cinnamon powder on top.
4. Serve warm or cold. Enjoy!

Cooking Tips:

- It is highly recommended to use rosewater in this rice pudding to experience a luxurious taste!
- If you want to have a delicious yellow rice pudding, add ⅓ teaspoon grounded saffron.

UC-related Tips:

- Always try to consume less sugar. Instead, you can use honey. If you cannot tolerate honey well, you can use maple syrup or stevia.

Nutrition Facts		
Servings: 6		
Amount per serving		
Calories		**290**
		% Daily Value*
Total Fat 5.7g		7%
Saturated Fat 1.3g		6%
Cholesterol 4mg		1%
Sodium 41mg		2%
Total Carbohydrate 55.3g		20%
Dietary Fiber 0.5g		2%
Total Sugars 27.7g		
Protein 5g		
Vitamin D 42mcg		211%
Calcium 134mg		10%
Iron 2mg		10%
Potassium 239mg		5%

GLUTEN-FREE APPLE PIE

This homemade gluten-free apple pie made with almond flour can satisfy you and your gut!

- Prep Time: 30 minutes
- Cook Time: 55 minutes
- Total Time: 85 minutes
- Serving: 6

Ingredients

- 1¾ cups almond flour, grounded
- ¼ cup tapioca flour+2 tablespoons tapioca flour
- 6 tablespoons extra virgin olive oil
- ½ large egg whisked
- 1 cup rolled oats or gluten-free oats
- 1 cup + ½ tablespoon coconut sugar or honey
- 1 teaspoon cinnamon powder
- ½ teaspoon ground ginger
- 4 apples, peeled, cored and sliced
- 1 tablespoon lemon juice
- 1 tablespoon vanilla extract
- Salt, to taste

Instructions

1. In a large bowl, mix almond and tapioca flour rolled oats and olive oil.
2. In a bowl, whisk egg a bit and adds ½ of an egg into the dough. Mix well to form a soft-ball. If the texture is not good, add 1 or 2 teaspoons of the whisked egg to the dough.
3. Put your dough on a parchment paper. Fridge the dough for an hour (Recommended keeping it in a fridge overnight).
4. Remove from the fridge. With a rolling pin, make a 10-12 inch disk. Then, gently move your dough disk to the pie plate. Return into its shape again if any part falls apart or breaks.
5. Crimp the edges with your fingertips. Make small holes in all parts of your dough.
6. In a large bowl, mix thinly sliced apples with lemon juice, vanilla extract, sugar or honey, ginger, and salt.
7. Cover your crust with the mix altogether.
8. Preheat oven to 400 °F.
9. Cover crust edges with a pie shield to avoid burning fast.
10. Bake for 15-20 minutes. Reduce heat to 350°F and let it bake for 40 minutes.
11. Remove from the oven. Cool down. Slice it and serve.

Cooking Tips:

- Cover the pie with aluminum foil if you see the toppings are getting brown so fast.

UC-related Tips:

- Make sure you can tolerate coconut sugar. Instead, you can use honey. If you cannot tolerate honey well, you can use maple syrup or stevia.

Nutrition Facts

Servings: 6

Amount per serving

Calories	380
	% Daily Value*
Total Fat 23.4g	30%
Saturated Fat 2.8g	14%
Cholesterol 14mg	5%
Sodium 18mg	1%
Total Carbohydrate 40.5g	15%
Dietary Fiber 6.1g	22%
Total Sugars 16.5g	
Protein 5.3g	
Vitamin D 1mcg	6%
Calcium 43mg	3%
Iron 2mg	10%
Potassium 299mg	6%

PUMPKIN PIE

Enjoy cooking a traditional pumpkin pie recipe for Ulcerative Colitis patients!

- Prep Time: 15 minutes
- Cook Time: 55 minutes
- Total Time: 70 minutes
- Serving: 4-6

<u>Ingredients</u>

- 2 cups pumpkin, peeled
- 1 ready pie crust, gluten-free (9-inch)
- 2 organic, free-range eggs
- 1.5 cups condensed milk or lactose-free condensed milk
- ½ teaspoon freshly grated ginger
- ½ teaspoon cinnamon powder
- ½ teaspoon salt

Instructions

1. Preheat oven to 400°F.
2. Blend the pumpkin with all other ingredients in a blender or whisk all ingredients in a large bowl.
3. Pour the mix in a ready crust and bake for 15 minutes.
4. Reduce heat to 350 °F and let it bake for 35-40 minutes. You can insert a fork into it. The fork has to come out very clean, showing that it perfectly cooked.
5. Serve and enjoy!

Cooking Tips:

- Cover the pie with aluminum foil if you see the toppings are getting brown so fast.

UC-related Tips:

- Make sure you can tolerate condensed milk. If you cannot, use lactose-free cow milk or almond milk instead.

Nutrition Facts

Servings: 6

Amount per serving	
Calories	**403**
	% Daily Value*
Total Fat 15.3g	20%
Saturated Fat 5.8g	29%
Cholesterol 81mg	27%
Sodium 258mg	11%
Total Carbohydrate 58.9g	21%
Dietary Fiber 2.8g	9%
Total Sugars 45.3g	
Protein 9.7g	
Vitamin D 5mcg	26%
Calcium 251mg	19%
Iron 2mg	11%
Potassium 497mg	11%

FRUIT DESSERT

A fresh cold fruit mix as a healthy dessert choice for Ulcerative Colitis patients.

- Prep Time: 20 minutes
- Total Time: 20 minutes
- Serving: 4

Ingredients

- 2 cups pineapple, cubed
- 2 cups cantaloupe, cubed
- 1 tablespoon maple syrup
- 3 tablespoons lime juice
- 1 cup papaya, cubed
- 2 cups honeydew melon, cubed

Instructions

1. In a large bowl, mix all ingredients.
2. Serve cold. Enjoy!

Cooking Tips:

- You can change the fruits in your fruit dessert as you wish, but make sure you can tolerate those fruits and always peel them off.
- You can mix your fruits with plain yogurt or lactose-free plain yogurt, as well.

UC-related Tips:

- Peel and poach fruits such as apple, pear, or peach if you want to add them into your fruit dessert.

Nutrition Facts

Servings: 4

Amount per serving

Calories **132**

	% Daily Value*
Total Fat 0.5g	1%
Saturated Fat 0.1g	1%
Cholesterol 0mg	0%
Sodium 33mg	1%
Total Carbohydrate 34g	12%
Dietary Fiber 3.3g	12%
Total Sugars 27.3g	
Protein 1.8g	
Vitamin D 0mcg	0%
Calcium 36mg	3%
Iron 1mg	4%
Potassium 594mg	13%

AVOCADO PEAR POPSICLE

Homemade popsicles are great desserts for people with UC. It is very easy to make popsicles at home. You need to try this recipe as an example:

- Prep Time: 10 minutes
- Freeze Time: 90 minutes
- Total Time: 100 minutes
- Serving: 4

Ingredients

- 2 avocados, peeled
- 2 pears, peeled and cored

Instructions

1. Blend well pears and avocados in a blender or food processor.
2. Fill up your Popsicle cups. Insert popsicle sticks and freeze.
3. Run the outside of the cup under hot water to remove the popsicles when you want to eat it.

Cooking Tips:

- You can change the fruit(s) in your popsicle as you wish, but make sure you can tolerate those fruits and always peel them off.

UC-related Tips:

- Peel and poach fruits such as apple, pear, or peach if you want to make a Popsicle from them.

Nutrition Facts

Servings: 4

Amount per serving

Calories	245
	% Daily Value*
Total Fat 19.7g	25%
Saturated Fat 4.1g	21%
Cholesterol 0mg	0%
Sodium 7mg	0%
Total Carbohydrate 19.2g	7%
Dietary Fiber 8.9g	32%
Total Sugars 7.3g	
Protein 2.2g	
Vitamin D 0mcg	0%
Calcium 18mg	1%
Iron 1mg	4%
Potassium 566mg	12%

LEMON SORBET

Try a Paleo-kind refreshing sorbet with great combinations of lemon juice and honey.

- Prep Time: 10 minutes
- Make Time: 120 minutes
- Total Time: 130 minutes
- Serving: 4

Ingredients

- 1 cup fresh lemon juice
- 2 tablespoons lemon zest
- 2 cups of water

- ½ cup honey or maple syrup
- 1 cup light cream
- ¼ teaspoon coconut extract

Instructions

1. In a medium pot, mix your honey (or maple syrup), lemon zest, and water until the honey dissolves and gets warm.
2. Add lemon juice or squeeze a lemon to the pot. Stir a bit.
3. Pour your sorbet mixture into a metal pan or pot or an ice cream maker.
4. Freeze for 2 hours. Scrape the sorbet with a spoon or fork every 15 minutes.
5. Enjoy!

Cooking Tips:

- You can change the fruit(s) in your sorbet as you wish, but make sure you can tolerate those fruits and always peel them off. Some fruits need to be cooked before making the sorbet.

UC-related Tips:

- Peel and poach fruits such as apple, pear, or peach if you want to make a sorbet from them.
- Make sure you can tolerate light cream. Instead, you can use almond milk. Be aware that it may need more freezing time if you use almond milk.

Nutrition Facts	
Servings: 4	
Amount per serving	
Calories	**234**
	% Daily Value*
Total Fat 9.8g	13%
Saturated Fat 6.3g	31%
Cholesterol 33mg	11%
Sodium 24mg	1%
Total Carbohydrate 37.7g	14%
Dietary Fiber 0.5g	2%
Total Sugars 36.3g	
Protein 1.3g	
Vitamin D 0mcg	0%
Calcium 29mg	2%
Iron 0mg	1%
Potassium 136mg	3%

MANGO ICE CREAM

This dairy-free mango ice cream is very easy to make. It is healthy and a tasty dessert choice for Ulcerative Colitis patients.

- Prep Time: 15 minutes
- Cook Time: 30 minutes
- Total Time: 45 minutes
- Serving: 6

Ingredients

- 1¾ cup coconut milk or almond milk
- 2 mangos, peeled
- ¼ cup honey or maple syrup
- ½ teaspoon vanilla extract

Instructions

1. Perfectly chill your coconut milk or almond milk in a fridge before you make this ice cream.
2. Blend milk, mango, maple syrup, and vanilla extract in a blender until perfectly smooth.

3. Pour your sorbet mixture into a metal container, pot, or an ice cream maker. If you use an ice cream maker, it takes about 30 minutes, but if you use a metal container, you may need to freeze it for 90-120 minutes.
4. Serve cold and enjoy it!

Cooking Tips:

- You can change the fruits in your ice cream as you desire, but make sure you can tolerate those fruits and always peel them off. Some fruits need to be cooked before making ice cream.

UC-related Tips:

- Peel and poach fruits such as apple, pear, or peach if you want to make a sorbet from them.
- Make sure you can tolerate coconut milk. Instead, you can use almond milk.

Nutrition Facts

Servings: 6

Amount per serving	
Calories	**272**
	% Daily Value*
Total Fat 17.1g	22%
Saturated Fat 14.8g	75%
Cholesterol 0mg	0%
Sodium 12mg	1%
Total Carbohydrate 32.3g	12%
Dietary Fiber 3.4g	12%
Total Sugars 29.3g	
Protein 2.6g	
Vitamin D 0mcg	0%
Calcium 24mg	2%
Iron 1mg	8%
Potassium 380mg	8%

SWEET POTATO PIE

If you want to make a pie with potato as a dessert, you can follow the recipe of sweet potato pie.

- Prep Time: 30 minutes
- Cook Time: 50 minutes
- Total Time: 80 minutes
- Serving: 4-6

Ingredients

- 2 medium sweet potatoes, peeled and cubed
- ¾ cup condensed milk or lactose-free condensed milk
- 1 deep-dish pie shell, uncooked (or gluten-free pastry shell)
- 2 tablespoons extra virgin olive oil
- ½ cup sugar or 1 tablespoon honey
- 2 large organic, free-range eggs
- 1 teaspoon vanilla extract
- ½ teaspoon cinnamon powder
- ½ teaspoon ground nutmeg
- ¼ teaspoon salt

Instructions

1. In a large pot, boil sweet potatoes by boiling water over medium heat.
2. Drain and mash potatoes by fork or blender.
3. Preheat oven to 400°F.
4. Mix mashed sweet potatoes with extra virgin olive oil, sugar, eggs, cinnamon, vanilla, nutmeg, and salt perfectly in a large bowl.
5. Pour the mix into a ready pie shell. Bake it for 20 minutes. Then, reduce heat around 350 °F and bake for 30-35 more minutes.
6. Serve warm or cold. Enjoy!

Cooking Tips:

- Cover the pie shell with aluminum foil if you see the toppings are getting brown so fast.

UC-related Tips:

- Make sure you can tolerate nutmeg. If you cannot, remove it from the ingredients.

Nutrition Facts	
Servings: 6	
Amount per serving	
Calories	**392**
	% Daily Value*
Total Fat 16.6g	21%
Saturated Fat 3.4g	17%
Cholesterol 75mg	25%
Sodium 74mg	3%
Total Carbohydrate 44.8g	16%
Dietary Fiber 1.1g	4%
Total Sugars 37.9g	
Protein 6.5g	
Vitamin D 6mcg	29%
Calcium 122mg	9%
Iron 1mg	3%
Potassium 370mg	8%

WHITE PANNA COTTA

A dairy-free, easy to make panna cotta for Ulcerative Colitis patients that comes with a lovely creamy taste of coconut milk.

- Prep Time: 10 minutes
- Chill time: 120 minutes
- Total Time: 130 minutes
- Serving: 4

Ingredients

- 1¾ cup coconut milk or almond milk
- ⅓ cup maple syrup or honey
- 2 teaspoons gelatin, grass-fed

- 1 teaspoon vanilla extract

Instructions

1. In a medium pan, heat coconut milk (or almond milk) and add gelatin. Stir until gelatin powder melts.
2. Add vanilla. Stir and let the mix get warmer for 3-5 minutes over medium heat until gelatin fully dissolved. Be aware that you should not boil the milk.
3. Remove from pan and add maple syrup or honey. Stir well.
4. Fill some small cups with the mixture and fridge it for 3-4 hours.
5. To remove Panna Cotta easily, put small cups in a hot water bowl for 2 minutes. Then, you can flip Panna Cottas on your dessert plates. Enjoy!

Cooking Tips:

- For having a fruity Panna Cotta, you can add poached and peeled fruit cubes in your mixture, as well.
- Alternatively, you can garnish your panna cotta with fruits you can tolerate.

UC-related Tips:

- Make sure you can tolerate coconut milk. If you cannot, use lactose-free cow milk or almond milk instead.

Nutrition Facts

Servings: 4

Amount per serving

Calories   **325**

	% Daily Value*
Total Fat 25.1g	32%
Saturated Fat 22.2g	111%
Cholesterol 0mg	0%
Sodium 25mg	1%
Total Carbohydrate 23.6g	9%
Dietary Fiber 2.3g	8%
Total Sugars 18.3g	
Protein 5.4g	
Vitamin D 0mcg	0%
Calcium 36mg	3%
Iron 2mg	12%
Potassium 332mg	7%

COCKTAILS AND SHAKES

BANANA MILKSHAKE

Enjoy tasting a traditional milkshake with banana.

- Prep Time: 5 minutes
- Serving: 1

Ingredients

- 1 banana
- 1 cup unsweetened almond or lactose-free milk
- ½ teaspoon stevia or two tablespoons honey or maple syrup

Instructions

- Blend all the above ingredients until smooth. Pour into a large glass. Enjoy!

Cooking Tips:

- You can use plain lactose-free yogurt or banana lactose-free yogurt instead of milk.

- Use agave syrup if you cannot tolerate maple syrup or honey.

<u>UC-related Tips:</u>

- Use honey only if you can tolerate it.

Nutrition Facts

Servings: 1

Amount per serving	
Calories	**145**
	% Daily Value*
Total Fat 3.9g	5%
Saturated Fat 0.4g	2%
Cholesterol 0mg	0%
Sodium 181mg	8%
Total Carbohydrate 29g	11%
Dietary Fiber 4.1g	15%
Total Sugars 14.4g	
Protein 2.3g	
Vitamin D 1mcg	7%
Calcium 306mg	24%
Iron 1mg	6%
Potassium 612mg	13%

COOLER DRINK

Enjoy tasting a great drink that makes you really cool!

- Prep Time: 5 minutes
- Serving: 1

<u>Ingredients</u>

- 2 cucumbers, peeled
- 10 mint leaves
- 1 cup lemon juice
- 1 cup of water
- Ice cubes

<u>Instructions</u>

- Blend all ingredients in a blender and then blend until smooth. Pour into a large glass. Enjoy!

Cooking Tips:

- You can add one teaspoon of freshly grated ginger to the drink as well.

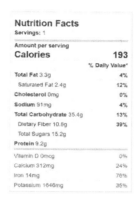

MANGO-BANANA SMOOTHIE

A great smoothie with mango and banana!

- Prep Time: 5 minutes
- Serving: 1-2

Ingredients

- 1 mango, diced
- 1 banana, diced
- 1 cup lactose-free milk or almond milk
- ½ teaspoon stevia (or honey or maple syrup)

Instructions

- Blend all ingredients in a blender and then blend until smooth. Pour into a large glass. Enjoy!

Cooking Tips:

- You can use plain lactose-free yogurt or banana lactose-free yogurt instead of milk for having a thick texture.
- Use agave syrup if you cannot tolerate maple syrup or honey.

UC-related Tips:

- Use honey only if you can tolerate it.
- If you cannot tolerate mango, use papaya instead.

Nutrition Facts

Servings: 2

Amount per serving

Calories 218

	% Daily Value*
Total Fat 3.4g	4%
Saturated Fat 1.7g	9%
Cholesterol 11mg	4%
Sodium 62mg	3%
Total Carbohydrate 44.7g	16%
Dietary Fiber 4.2g	15%
Total Sugars 30.2g	
Protein 6.3g	
Vitamin D 50mcg	250%
Calcium 171mg	13%
Iron 0mg	2%
Potassium 703mg	15%

GINGER COOL DRINK

A great healthy drink for Ulcerative Colitis patients.

- Prep Time: 5 minutes
- Serving: 1

Ingredients

- 5 tablespoons applesauce
- 1 cup of water
- 1 cup of cooked pear or 1 can of pear compote
- 1 small piece of ginger or 2 teaspoons ginger powder

Instructions

- Blend all ingredients in a blender and then blend until smooth. Pour into a large glass. Enjoy!

Cooking Tips:

- You can use lactose-free milk or almond milk instead of water to make a great smoothie.
- You can add honey (if you can tolerate) or ½ tablespoon of stevia for sweetness.

Nutrition Facts

Servings: 1

Amount per serving

Calories	138
	% Daily Value*
Total Fat 0.5g	1%
Saturated Fat 0.1g	0%
Cholesterol 0mg	0%
Sodium 5mg	0%
Total Carbohydrate 35.7g	13%
Dietary Fiber 6.4g	23%
Total Sugars 23.5g	
Protein 1g	
Vitamin D 0mcg	0%
Calcium 21mg	2%
Iron 1mg	4%
Potassium 292mg	6%

AVOCADO SMOOTHIE

A great healthy drink for Ulcerative Colitis patients with healthy fats. If you like, you can add protein powder in the smoothie.

- Prep Time: 5 minutes
- Serving: 1-2

Ingredients

- 1 avocado
- 1 banana

- 1 cup lactose-free milk or unsweetened almond milk
- 2 tablespoons maple syrup or 1 teaspoon stevia

Instructions

- Blend all ingredients in a blender and then blend until smooth. Pour into a large glass. Enjoy!

Cooking Tips:

- Use can use honey (if you can tolerate) instead of maple syrup.

Nutrition Facts

Servings: 2

Amount per serving

Calories	375
	% Daily Value*
Total Fat 22.3g	29%
Saturated Fat 5.7g	29%
Cholesterol 10mg	3%
Sodium 71mg	3%
Total Carbohydrate 42g	15%
Dietary Fiber 6.3g	36%
Total Sugars 25.8g	
Protein 6.6g	
Vitamin D 0mcg	0%
Calcium 178mg	14%
Iron 1mg	6%
Potassium 739mg	16%

BANANA-CINNAMON SMOOTHIE

A classical thick smoothie to enjoy!

- Prep Time: 5 minutes
- Serving: 1

Ingredients

- 1 banana
- 1 cup vanilla yogurt or lactose-free yogurt
- 2 teaspoons maple syrup or ½ teaspoon stevia
- 1 teaspoon cinnamon

- ⅓ cup of ice

Instructions

- Blend all ingredients in a blender and then blend until smooth. Pour into a large glass. Enjoy!

Cooking Tips:

- Use can use honey (if you can tolerate) instead of maple syrup.
- Plain yogurt can also be used instead of vanilla yogurt.

Nutrition Facts
Servings: 1

Amount per serving

Calories	320
	% Daily Value*
Total Fat 3.5g	4%
Saturated Fat 2.6g	13%
Cholesterol 15mg	5%
Sodium 174mg	8%
Total Carbohydrate 55g	20%
Dietary Fiber 4.3g	15%
Total Sugars 39.7g	
Protein 15.3g	
Vitamin D 0mcg	0%
Calcium 466mg	37%
Iron 1mg	5%
Potassium 1033mg	22%

PEACH-MANGO-BANANA SMOOTHIE

A fabulous smoothie with three different fruits to enjoy!

- Prep Time: 5 minutes
- Serving: 1-2

Ingredients

- ½ mango, diced
- ½ banana, diced
- 1 peach, diced and skin-removed

- 1 cup plain yogurt or lactose-free yogurt
- ½ cup of ice
- 1 teaspoon stevia (or honey or maple syrup)

Instructions

- Blend all ingredients in a blender and then blend until smooth. Pour into a large glass. Enjoy!

Cooking Tips:

- You can use two tablespoons of agave syrup, honey, or sugar instead of stevia if you can tolerate it.

UC-related Tips:

- Use honey only if you can tolerate it.
- If you cannot tolerate mango, use papaya instead.

Nutrition Facts	
Servings: 1	
Amount per serving	
Calories	**387**
	% Daily Value*
Total Fat 4.2g	5%
Saturated Fat 2.7g	13%
Cholesterol 15mg	5%
Sodium 174mg	8%
Total Carbohydrate 69.9g	25%
Dietary Fiber 6.5g	23%
Total Sugars 61.4g	
Protein 17.4g	
Vitamin D 0mcg	0%
Calcium 470mg	36%
Iron 1mg	5%
Potassium 1352mg	29%

PEACH-GINGER SMOOTHIE

A ginger-based smoothie with a fantastic taste!

- Prep Time: 5 minutes
- Serving: 1

Ingredients

- 1 peach, diced and skin-removed
- 1 cup lactose-free milk or unsweetened almond milk
- 1 tablespoon fresh grated ginger
- 1 teaspoon stevia (or one tablespoon honey or maple syrup)

Instructions

- Blend all ingredients in a blender and then blend until smooth. Pour into a large glass. Enjoy!

Cooking Tips:

- You can use two tablespoons of agave syrup, honey, or sugar instead of stevia if you can tolerate it.

UC-related Tips:

- Use honey only if you can tolerate it.

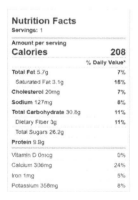

Nutrition Facts	
Servings: 1	
Amount per serving	
Calories	**208**
	% Daily Value*
Total Fat 5.7g	7%
Saturated Fat 3.1g	16%
Cholesterol 20mg	7%
Sodium 127mg	6%
Total Carbohydrate 30.8g	11%
Dietary Fiber 3g	11%
Total Sugars 26.2g	
Protein 9.8g	
Vitamin D 0mcg	0%
Calcium 306mg	24%
Iron 1mg	5%
Potassium 358mg	8%

POMEGRANATE-ANGELICA SMOOTHIE

Enjoy a healthy smoothie with a fantastic sour taste!

- Prep Time: 5 minutes
- Serving: 1-2

Ingredients

- 1 cup pomegranate juice
- ½ cup plain yogurt or lactose-free yogurt
- 1 tablespoon Angelica root powder (optional)
- 1 teaspoon salt

Instructions

- Blend all ingredients in a blender and then blend until smooth. Pour into a large glass. Enjoy!

Cooking Tips:

- You can use one tablespoon of honey or maple syrup for giving sweetness to the smoothie if you can tolerate it.

UC-related Tips:

- Use honey only if you can tolerate it.
- Make sure you are not eating pomegranate seeds.

Nutrition Facts

Servings: 1

Amount per serving

Calories	237
	% Daily Value*
Total Fat 1.5g	2%
Saturated Fat 1.2g	6%
Cholesterol 7mg	2%
Sodium 2421mg	105%
Total Carbohydrate 45.6g	17%
Dietary Fiber 0g	0%
Total Sugars 40.6g	
Protein 7g	
Vitamin D 0mcg	0%
Calcium 246mg	19%
Iron 0mg	1%
Potassium 887mg	19%

APPLE-GINGER SMOOTHIE

A ginger-based smoothie with a fantastic taste!

- Prep Time: 5 minutes
- Serving: 1-2

Ingredients

- 1 apple, diced and skin-removed
- 1 cup lactose-free milk or unsweetened almond milk
- 3 tablespoons lime juice
- 1 tablespoon fresh grated ginger
- 1 tablespoon honey

Instructions

- Blend all ingredients in a blender and then blend until smooth. Pour into a large glass. Enjoy!

Cooking Tips:

- You can use one tablespoon of maple syrup, or one teaspoon of stevia instead of honey.

UC-related Tips:

- Use honey only if you can tolerate it.

Nutrition Facts

Servings: 1

Amount per serving

Calories   **345**

	% Daily Value*
Total Fat 5.8g	7%
Saturated Fat 3.1g	16%
Cholesterol 20mg	7%
Sodium 131mg	6%
Total Carbohydrate 70.5g	26%
Dietary Fiber 6.4g	23%
Total Sugars 53.7g	
Protein 9.4g	
Vitamin D 0mcg	0%
Calcium 318mg	24%
Iron 2mg	10%
Potassium 399mg	8%

BLOODY RED DRINK!

Enjoy a healthy drink with an amazing sour taste!

- Prep Time: 5 minutes
- Serving: 1-2

Ingredients

- 1 cup pomegranate juice
- ½ beet juice
- ½ tablespoon Angelica powder
- 1 teaspoon salt
- 1 tablespoon honey (or maple syrup), to taste

Instructions

- Blend all the ingredients in a blender until smooth. Pour into a large glass. Enjoy!

Cooking Tips:

- You can use one teaspoon of stevia instead of honey or maple syrup.

UC-related Tips:

- If you are experiencing a flare-up, remove the beet from the recipe.
- Use honey only if you can tolerate it.

Nutrition Facts

Servings: 1

Amount per serving

Calories	267
	% Daily Value*
Total Fat 0g	0%
Saturated Fat 0g	0%
Cholesterol 0mg	0%
Sodium 2384mg	104%
Total Carbohydrate 66.3g	24%
Dietary Fiber 0g	0%
Total Sugars 60.3g	
Protein 1.6g	
Vitamin D 0mcg	0%
Calcium 23mg	2%
Iron 0mg	1%
Potassium 611mg	13%

PINEAPPLE-MANGO SMOOTHIE

Enjoy a great combination of pineapple and mango in a refreshing smoothie!

- Prep Time: 5-7 minutes
- Serving: 2

Ingredients

- 1 cup mango, diced
- 1 cup pineapple chunks
- 1 cup almond or lactose-free milk
- 1 tablespoon honey or maple syrup

Instructions

- Blend all ingredients in a blender and then blend until smooth. Pour into a large glass. Enjoy!

Cooking Tips:

- You can use one teaspoon of stevia instead of honey or maple syrup.
- If you can tolerate, you can use coconut milk instead of almond or lactose-free milk

UC-related Tips:

- Use honey only if you can tolerate it.
- If mango irritates your gut, use papaya instead.

Nutrition Facts

Servings: 2

Amount per serving

Calories	398
	% Daily Value*
Total Fat 29g	37%
Saturated Fat 25.5g	127%
Cholesterol 0mg	0%
Sodium 20mg	1%
Total Carbohydrate 38.5g	14%
Dietary Fiber 5.1g	18%
Total Sugars 32g	
Protein 3.9g	
Vitamin D 0mcg	0%
Calcium 38mg	3%
Iron 2mg	13%
Potassium 550mg	12%

CANTALOUPE SMOOTHIE

Enjoy a great smoothie with cantaloupe!

- Prep Time: 5 minutes
- Serving: 1-2

Ingredients

- 1 cup cantaloupe, diced
- ½ cup vanilla yogurt or lactose-free yogurt
- ½ cup of orange juice
- 1 tablespoon honey (or maple syrup), to taste
- 2 ice cubes

Instructions

- Blend all ingredients in a blender and then blend until smooth. Pour into a large glass. Enjoy!

Cooking Tips:

- You can use 1 teaspoon of stevia instead of honey or maple syrup.

UC-related Tips:

- Use honey only if you can tolerate it.
- If orange juice irritates your gut, simply remove it from the recipe.

Nutrition Facts
Servings: 1

Amount per serving	
Calories	**260**
	% Daily Value*
Total Fat 2.1g	3%
Saturated Fat 1.4g	7%
Cholesterol 7mg	2%
Sodium 113mg	5%
Total Carbohydrate 51.6g	19%
Dietary Fiber 1.7g	6%
Total Sugars 48.5g	
Protein 9.2g	
Vitamin D 0mcg	0%
Calcium 241mg	18%
Iron 2mg	11%
Potassium 962mg	20%

CANTALOUPE-MIX SMOOTHIE

Enjoy a great mix of cantaloupe with mango, lemon, and orange!

- Prep Time: 5-10 minutes
- Serving: 2

Ingredients

- 1 cup cantaloupe, diced
- ½ cup mango, diced
- ½ cup almond milk or lactose-free cow milk
- ½ cup of orange juice
- 2 tablespoons lemon
- 1 tablespoon honey (or maple syrup), to taste
- 2 ice cubes

Instructions

- Blend the ingredients in a blender until smooth. Pour into a large glass. Enjoy!

Cooking Tips:

- You can use one teaspoon of stevia instead of honey or maple syrup.

UC-related Tips:

- Use honey only if you can tolerate it.
- If orange juice irritates your gut, remove it from the recipe.
- If you cannot tolerate mango, use papaya instead.

Nutrition Facts

Servings: 2

Amount per serving

Calories	253
	% Daily Value*
Total Fat 14.8g	19%
Saturated Fat 12.8g	64%
Cholesterol 0mg	0%
Sodium 23mg	1%
Total Carbohydrate 32.2g	12%
Dietary Fiber 3.2g	11%
Total Sugars 27.9g	
Protein 3g	
Vitamin D 0mcg	0%
Calcium 26mg	2%
Iron 2mg	12%
Potassium 583mg	12%

APPLESAUCE-AVOCADO SMOOTHIE

Have you tried the taste of applesauce with avocado? Try this smoothie cold!

- Prep Time: 5-7 minutes
- Serving: 1

Ingredients

- 1 cup unsweetened almond or lactose-free milk
- ½ avocado
- ½ cup applesauce
- ¼ teaspoon ground cinnamon
- ½ cup ice

Instructions

- Blend all ingredients in a blender. Blend the mix until smooth. Pour into a large glass. Enjoy!

Cooking Tips:

- You can use ½ teaspoon of stevia or 1 tablespoon of honey for sweetness.

Nutrition Facts	
Servings: 1	
Amount per serving	
Calories	**299**
	% Daily Value*
Total Fat 23.2g	30%
Saturated Fat 4.4g	22%
Cholesterol 0mg	0%
Sodium 189mg	8%
Total Carbohydrate 24.9g	9%
Dietary Fiber 9.5g	34%
Total Sugars 12.8g	
Protein 3.1g	
Vitamin D 1mcg	7%
Calcium 322mg	25%
Iron 2mg	8%
Potassium 771mg	16%

PINA COLADA SMOOTHIE

A classical gluten-free Mexican smoothie for your parties!

- Prep Time: 5 minutes
- Serving: 1

Ingredients

- 1 cup pineapple chunks
- ½ cup unsweetened almond milk or lactose-free milk
- 1 banana
- ½ teaspoon coconut extract, to taste
- 1 tablespoon honey, maple syrup or one teaspoon stevia (optional)
- ¼ cup shredded coconut (optional)

Instructions

- Blend all ingredients in a blender and then blend until smooth and creamy. Pour into a large glass. Enjoy!

Cooking Tips:

- For sweetness, you can add stevia, honey, or maple syrup as instructed.

UC-related Tips:

- Use honey only if you can tolerate it.
- Do not use coconut extract if you are experiencing a flare-up.

Nutrition Facts

Servings: 1

Amount per serving

Calories   **348**

	% Daily Value*
Total Fat 9g	12%
Saturated Fat 6.2g	31%
Cholesterol 0mg	0%
Sodium 98mg	4%
Total Carbohydrate 70.2g	26%
Dietary Fiber 7.7g	28%
Total Sugars 49.4g	
Protein 3.4g	
Vitamin D 1mcg	3%
Calcium 179mg	14%
Iron 4mg	22%
Potassium 783mg	17%

SNACKS

DICED FRUITS

You can dice fresh fruits you can tolerate and use them between your daily main meals. Papaya, honeydew melon, cantaloupe, pineapple, and banana are some of the best fruits for Ulcerative Colitis patients.

PLAIN YOGURT WITH POACHED FRUITS

Another great snack is mixing plain/vanilla yogurt or lactose-free plain or vanilla yogurt with fruits you can tolerate or peeled and poached fruits. As explained, papaya, honeydew melon, cantaloupe, pineapple, and banana are some of the best fruits for Ulcerative Colitis patients. The following recipe shows how to poach fruits like apple and peach to make a delicious homemade compote.

POACHED FRUIT COMPOTE

It is a great choice that can be consumed by Ulcerative Colitis patients.

- Prep Time: 10 minutes

- Cook Time: 40 Minutes
- Total Time: 50 minutes
- Serving: 6

Ingredients

- 4 peaches, skin removed and thinly sliced
- 1 lb apple, pitted and skin removed
- 1 teaspoon cinnamon powder
- 1 cup honey or maple syrup
- 1 teaspoon vanilla extract

Instructions

1. In a large pot, cook fruits in boiling water over medium heat until softened.
2. In a large bowl, mix well all ingredients (except fruits) together.
3. Pour the syrup over fruits and let the compote be thickened.
4. Pour compote into a jar. Serve hot or cold. Enjoy!

Cooking Tips:

- You can poach fruits with the skin and remove the skin after poaching and before adding syrup to it.
- If you can tolerate sugar and for better sweetness, you can use ½ cup of cane sugar.
- You can poach other fruits such as pear with the same instructions.

UC-related Tips:

- Make sure you wash fruits thoroughly after peeling them off.

- Some Ulcerative Colitis patients cannot tolerate peach. Always make and consume poached fruits you can tolerate.

Nutrition Facts	
Servings: 6	
Amount per serving	
Calories	**232**
	% Daily Value*
Total Fat 0.3g	0%
Saturated Fat 0g	0%
Cholesterol 0mg	0%
Sodium 3mg	0%
Total Carbohydrate 61.1g	22%
Dietary Fiber 2.5g	9%
Total Sugars 59.7g	
Protein 1.2g	
Vitamin D 0mcg	0%
Calcium 4mg	0%
Iron 1mg	4%
Potassium 260mg	6%

APPLESAUCE

Applesauce is a fantastic option for people who live with Ulcerative Colitis. You can purchase applesauce from different stores. It is recommended to use organic applesauce, or you can make it at home:

HOMEMADE APPLESAUCE

- Prep Time: 10 minutes
- Cook Time: 30 Minutes
- Total Time: 40 minutes
- Serving: 4

Ingredients

- 6 organic apples, peeled, cored and cubed
- ½ cup boiling water
- ½ teaspoon cinnamon powder
- ¼ cup sugar or four tablespoons honey
- 2 tablespoons fresh lemon juice

- ¼ teaspoon salt

Instructions

1. In a large pot, cook apples with boiling water, lemon juice, cinnamon, sugar or honey, and salt over medium-low heat until softened. Remove from heat.
2. You can mash all ingredients by using a fork or blend with a blender or a food processor.
3. Pour applesauce into a suitable container or jar. Serve warm or cold. Enjoy!

Cooking Tips:

- Pink lady apples are preferable for making delicious applesauce.

UC-related Tips:

- Make sure you wash apples thoroughly after peeling them off.
- If you cannot tolerate sugar or honey well, you may add one tablespoon of Stevia instead.

Nutrition Facts

Servings: 4

Amount per serving

Calories 223

	% Daily Value*
Total Fat 0.7g	1%
Saturated Fat 0.1g	0%
Cholesterol 0mg	0%
Sodium 5mg	0%
Total Carbohydrate 58.9g	21%
Dietary Fiber 8.1g	29%
Total Sugars 47.5g	
Protein 1g	
Vitamin D 0mcg	0%
Calcium 3mg	0%
Iron 2mg	8%
Potassium 368mg	8%

AVOCADO DIP

A modified avocado dip recipe is a great snack candidate for Ulcerative Colitis patients.

- Prep Time: 5 minutes
- Cook Time: 0 minutes
- Total Time: 5 minutes
- Serving: 4-6

Ingredients

- 6 avocados, peeled
- ½ tablespoon extra virgin olive oil
- ¼ cup chopped fresh cilantro
- 2 tablespoons fresh lime juice
- 1 teaspoon fresh lemon juice
- ½ teaspoon salt

Instructions

1. In a large bowl, mash avocados with a fork.
2. Add extra virgin olive oil and other ingredients into it.
3. Enjoy!

Cooking Tips:

- You can serve guacamole with tacos if you can tolerate it.
- If you can tolerate a few tomatoes and onions, cube them and then add them into your guacamole.

UC-related Tips:

- Do not use fresh cilantro if you are experiencing a severe flare-up. Do not take taco chips, as well.

Nutrition Facts

Servings: 6

Amount per serving

Calories 422

	% Daily Value*
Total Fat 40.4g	52%
Saturated Fat 8.4g	42%
Cholesterol 0mg	0%
Sodium 207mg	9%
Total Carbohydrate 18g	7%
Dietary Fiber 13.5g	48%
Total Sugars 1.2g	
Protein 3.9g	
Vitamin D 0mcg	0%
Calcium 26mg	2%
Iron 1mg	7%
Potassium 988mg	21%

HOMEMADE HUMMUS

A healthy and tasty middle-eastern snack. An excellent option for vegetarians and Ulcerative Colitis patients during the remission period.

- Prep Time: 5 minutes
- Cook Time: 60 minutes
- Total Time: 65 minutes
- Serving: 4

Ingredients

- ¼ lb dried chickpeas (soaked in water for one night)
- 1½ tablespoon tahini
- 1 tablespoon lemon juice
- 2 tablespoons extra virgin olive oil, divided
- ¼ teaspoon cumin
- ½ teaspoon salt
- 1 tablespoon water
- 1 teaspoon baking soda (optional)
- 1 teaspoon paprika powder (optional)
- ½ teaspoon garlic powder (optional)

Instructions

1. First, Ulcerative Colitis patients need to soak the chickpeas overnight in water and optionally add baking soda to the water.
2. Cook your chickpeas in a large pot with water, over medium heat for about one hour. Check if chickpeas cooked well by crushing one of them with a fork in your hand.
3. When chickpeas cooked, drain them and put them in a blender.
4. Add 1 tablespoon of extra virgin olive oil, lemon juice, tahini, cumin powder, salt, and garlic powder (optional) to the blender. Blend until your hummus gets a soft, creamy texture equally.
5. Sprinkle with one tablespoon extra virgin olive oil or paprika powder (optional).
6. Serve immediately or fridge it.

Cooking Tips:

- Hummus is well-matched with white pita bread.
- You can serve hummus, hot or cold.

UC-related Tips:

- Do not use paprika and garlic powders in hummus if you are experiencing a severe flare-up.
- Eat hummus in moderation when you are in remission. It is better to avoid making Hummus during flares, or make and eat a little bit of it.

Nutrition Facts		
Servings: 4		
Amount per serving		
Calories		**198**
		% Daily Value*
Total Fat 11.8g		15%
Saturated Fat 1.6g		8%
Cholesterol 0mg		0%
Sodium 305mg		13%
Total Carbohydrate 18.5g		7%
Dietary Fiber 5.5g		20%
Total Sugars 3.1g		
Protein 6.5g		
Vitamin D 0mcg		0%
Calcium 56mg		4%
Iron 2mg		13%
Potassium 279mg		6%

TOFU

Tofu is a fantastic snack option for Ulcerative Colitis patients. It is based on soy milk and is rich in calcium and Iron, needed for most Ulcerative Colitis patients. Here is a sample recipe of a snack with Tofu:

AVOCADO TOFU TOAST

Enjoy a healthy and rich daily snack!

- Prep Time: 10 minutes
- Cook Time: 35 minutes
- Total Time: 45 minutes
- Serving: 4

Ingredients

- 1½ cup firm tofu, pressed and drained
- 1 avocado, cubed
- 1 tablespoon extra virgin olive oil
- ½ teaspoon garlic powder (optional)
- Salt and pepper, to taste

Instructions

1. Preheat your oven to 400 °F.
2. Choose a baking sheet, cover it with parchment paper or spray extra virgin olive oil. Cut tofu-like cubes of 1.5 inches and spray extra virgin olive oil on it.
3. Let it bake for 15 minutes until golden brown and crispy. Flip tofu and cook for another 10 minutes. Remove from the oven. Let it rest for 10 minutes.
4. Cube avocado on a plate and add garlic powder (optional), salt, and pepper.
5. Mix the tofu with avocado in a bowl. Enjoy!

Cooking Tips:

- You may want to add one tablespoon of lemon juice to create another great taste.

UC-related Tips:

- Do not use pepper and garlic powder in this toast if you are experiencing a flare-up.

Nutrition Facts	
Servings: 4	
Amount per serving	
Calories	**199**
	% Daily Value*
Total Fat 17.2g	22%
Saturated Fat 3.4g	17%
Cholesterol 0mg	0%
Sodium 14mg	1%
Total Carbohydrate 5.9g	2%
Dietary Fiber 4.2g	15%
Total Sugars 0.8g	
Protein 8.7g	
Vitamin D 0mcg	0%
Calcium 196mg	15%
Iron 2mg	10%
Potassium 384mg	8%

ALMOND BUTTER SANDWICH

Almond butter is a fantastic source of fiber and magnesium for Ulcerative Colitis patients. It is recommended to use smooth almond butter.

- Prep Time: 5 minutes
- Total Time: 5 minutes
- Serving: 1

Ingredients

- 2 slices of white bread or white gluten-free bread
- 1 tablespoon organic smooth almond butter

Instructions

1. Spread one piece of bread with almond butter.
2. Toast and enjoy!

Cooking Tips:

- You can combine the almond butter sandwich with almond milk or lactose-free cow milk perfectly.

UC-related Tips:

- Remember to use smooth almond butter if you have large intestinal strictures due to Ulcerative Colitis.

Nutrition Facts

Servings: 1

Amount per serving

Calories 313

	% Daily Value*
Total Fat 17.7g	23%
Saturated Fat 1.9g	9%
Cholesterol 0mg	0%
Sodium 341mg	15%
Total Carbohydrate 32.3g	12%
Dietary Fiber 5.2g	19%
Total Sugars 4.2g	
Protein 8.8g	
Vitamin D 0mcg	0%
Calcium 156mg	12%
Iron 3mg	16%
Potassium 280mg	6%

GLUTEN-FREE MUFFINS

You may eat different types of muffins, but you have to make sure about the ingredients. The muffin should not be made with fruits you cannot tolerate. Moreover, try not to eat muffins that are made with whole wheat flour. If you are gluten-intolerant or suffering from UC, you can make your muffins at home:

- Prep Time: 15 minutes
- Cook Time: 45 minutes
- Total Time: 60 minutes
- Serving: 5-10 (10 Muffins)

Ingredients

- 2 tablespoons extra virgin olive oil or avocado oil
- 2½ cups almond flour, blanched
- 3 large organic free-range eggs
- ¼ cup organic maple syrup
- 2 teaspoons vanilla extract
- ¼ cup banana, mashed
- 1 teaspoon lemon juice
- ¾ teaspoon baking soda

- ¼ teaspoon cinnamon powder
- ½ teaspoon salt

Instructions

1. Preheat your oven to 375 °F.
2. In a large bowl, mix almond flour, cinnamon, baking soda, and salt. Whisk well.
3. In another bowl, add extra virgin olive oil, vanilla extract, eggs, ripe banana, maple syrup, and lemon juice. Whisk well.
4. Mix the two bowls and stir well with a wooden spoon until flour mixed well with other ingredients.
5. Prepare ten muffin cups. Pour them to the top and then bake for 15 minutes.
6. To avoid browning quickly, loosely cover muffins with an aluminum foil. Cook for another 15 minutes.
7. Put a toothpick in a muffin to check if it cooks well or not. If cooked well, the toothpick should not stick to the muffin.
8. Remove from the oven. Let the muffins cool for 15 more minutes. Enjoy!

Cooking Tips:

- You need to use finely grounded skin removed flour.

UC-related Tips:

- During a flare-up, try not to use coconut oil a lot.

Nutrition Facts

Servings: 10

Amount per serving

Calories	366
	% Daily Value*
Total Fat 30.7g	39%
Saturated Fat 2.9g	14%
Cholesterol 65mg	22%
Sodium 242mg	11%
Total Carbohydrate 16.1g	6%
Dietary Fiber 5.1g	18%
Total Sugars 7.8g	
Protein 12.8g	
Vitamin D 0mcg	0%
Calcium 132mg	10%
Iron 2mg	11%
Potassium 31mg	1%

CHEESE STICKS

Cheese sticks are excellent sources of calcium. If you are in remission, you may consume cheese sticks as snacks. Remember to choose low fat or fat-free options. If you are lactose-intolerant, you may use lactose-free Swiss, Havarti, or aged cheddar. One cheddar cheese sticks have the following nutrition fact:

Nutrition Facts

Servings: 1

Amount per serving

Calories	110
	% Daily Value*
Total Fat 9g	12%
Saturated Fat 5g	25%
Cholesterol 30mg	10%
Sodium 180mg	8%
Total Carbohydrate 0g	0%
Dietary Fiber 0g	0%
Total Sugars 0g	
Protein 7g	
Vitamin D 0mcg	0%
Calcium 200mg	15%
Iron 0mg	0%
Potassium 0mg	0%

AVOCADO TUNA TOAST

A very fast sandwich you can prepare at home.

- Prep Time: 10 minutes

- Cook Time: 0 minutes
- Total Time: 10 minutes
- Serving: 4

Ingredients

- 2 avocados
- 2 tablespoons organic low-fat mayonnaise
- 1 teaspoon cumin powder
- 1 can of tuna in olive oil or water
- ¼ cup apple, chopped and peeled off
- 4 white toasts or any gluten-free bread
- Salt to taste
- 1 teaspoon Dijon mustard (optional)
- Pepper to taste (optional)

Instructions

1. Choose a small bowl. Mix tuna with smashed avocado with mayo, cumin powder, peeled off apple (cut into small pieces), mustard (optional), salt, and pepper (optional).
2. Place tuna mix on two toast slices. Cover with other slices.
3. Toast and enjoy!

Cooking Tips:

- You can make this sandwich without mayonnaise sauce, as well.

UC-related Tips:

- Do not use black pepper, cumin powder, or mustard if you are experiencing a flare-up.

Nutrition Facts

Servings: 4

Amount per serving

Calories 386

	% Daily Value*
Total Fat 26.7g	34%
Saturated Fat 5.2g	26%
Cholesterol 17mg	6%
Sodium 268mg	12%
Total Carbohydrate 23.3g	8%
Dietary Fiber 7.7g	27%
Total Sugars 3g	
Protein 15.8g	
Vitamin D 0mcg	0%
Calcium 45mg	3%
Iron 2mg	11%
Potassium 689mg	15%

RICE CRACKERS

Most rice crackers in the market are gluten-free and tasty snacks for Ulcerative Colitis patients. White rice is an excellent carbohydrate for people with UC.

GLUTEN-FREE RICE CRACKER

A great example of making a rice cracker as a snack.

- Prep Time: 10 minutes
- Cook Time: 15 minutes
- Total Time: 25 minutes
- Serving: 6

Ingredients

- 1 cup white rice flour
- 2 tablespoons extra virgin olive oil
- ⅓ cup of water
- ½ tablespoon salt
- 1 teaspoon honey (optional)

Instructions

1. Preheat oven to 350 °F.

2. In a large bowl, mix white rice flour with oil, salt, honey, and water to create a smooth dough.
3. Roll out the dough on a floured surface and make round, thin rice cookies.
4. Make holes throughout rice cookies by using a fork. Spray them with extra virgin olive oil.
5. Bake crackers for about 15 minutes until slightly golden. Enjoy!

Cooking Tips:

- You can make this cracker in a large pan, as well. Just bake them with extra virgin olive oil over low heat until golden both sides.

UC-related Tips:

- Make sure you are using white rice flour and no other types of rice flours such as brown rice flours.

Nutrition Facts

Servings: 6

Amount per serving

Calories 190

	% Daily Value*
Total Fat 5.2g	7%
Saturated Fat 0.7g	3%
Cholesterol 0mg	0%
Sodium 582mg	25%
Total Carbohydrate 32g	12%
Dietary Fiber 1g	4%
Total Sugars 0g	
Protein 2g	
Vitamin D 0mcg	0%
Calcium 1mg	0%
Iron 0mg	0%
Potassium 0mg	0%

GINGER BISCUITS

Ginger is rich in potassium and vitamin B6 with excellent anti-inflammatory properties. Hence, ginger-based snacks are great snack options for Ulcerative Colitis patients.

GLUTEN-FREE GINGER BISCUITS

Enjoy making a gluten-free, dairy-free ginger biscuit in your home, perfectly matched to UC conditions.

- Prep Time: 15 minutes
- Cook Time: 20 minutes
- Total Time: 35 minutes
- Serving: 4-6

Ingredients

- ¾ cup shortening or half a cup + 1 tablespoon extra virgin olive oil
- 2 cups gluten-free flour or grated almond flour
- 2 tablespoons honey
- 1 organic, free-range egg
- 2 teaspoons baking soda
- ¼ cup molasses
- 1½ teaspoons freshly grated ginger
- 1 teaspoon cinnamon powder
- ½ teaspoon salt

Instructions

1. In a large bowl, mix oil (or shortening), sugar, molasses, and egg.
2. In another large bowl, mix flour, ginger, baking soda, cinnamon, and salt.
3. Slowly combine ingredients of both bowls until making a soft dough.
4. Let the dough rest for 45 minutes.
5. Preheat oven to 375°F.
6. Roll the dough and make 2-inch (5cm) balls. Pour honey on dough balls.

7. Use cookie sheets with parchment paper. Put balls on cooking sheets and bake for 12-15 minutes until seeing cracks and until having a light brown color.
8. Remove from the oven and cool biscuits for five minutes. Enjoy!

Cooking Tips:

- Shortening gives you a better ginger biscuit texture. However, Ulcerative Colitis patients may not tolerate it well. Alternatively, use olive oil.
- If you cannot tolerate honey, you can use a little bit of sugar or maple syrup.
- You can substitute ¼ cup of molasses with ¼ cup maple syrup.

UC-related Tips:

- Do not use molasses if you cannot tolerate it. Instead, use maple syrup.

Nutrition Facts	
Servings: 6	
Amount per serving	
Calories	**367**
	% Daily Value*
Total Fat 4.5g	6%
Saturated Fat 1.1g	5%
Cholesterol 27mg	9%
Sodium 660mg	29%
Total Carbohydrate 77.2g	28%
Dietary Fiber 8.5g	30%
Total Sugars 15.3g	
Protein 5.8g	
Vitamin D 3mcg	13%
Calcium 34mg	3%
Iron 1mg	6%
Potassium 236mg	5%

ZUCCHINI CHIPS

Zucchini chips are a healthy, low-calorie snack for Ulcerative Colitis patients with lots of crunchiness as well as vitamin C and B6!

- Prep Time: 20 minutes
- Cook Time: 90 minutes
- Total Time: 110 minutes
- Serving: 2-4

Ingredients

- 2 zucchinis, sliced thin
- 1 tablespoon extra virgin olive oil
- Salt, to taste
- ¼ teaspoon cumin powder (optional)
- ½ teaspoon garlic powder (optional)

Instructions

1- Slice zucchinis lengthwise and thin by a slicer.
2- Take out the moisture from zucchinis using clean paper towels. Hold and press down paper towels on zucchinis.
3- Preheat the over to 250 °F.
4- Spray olive oil on parchment papers and then, place zucchinis on them.
5- Spray or pour olive oil on top of zucchinis as well. Sprinkle salt, cumin powder (optional) and garlic powder (optional).
6- Bake zucchinis for about 80-90 minutes until golden.
7- Remove from the oven. Dry zucchinis with a paper towel. Enjoy!

Cooking Tips:

- You can also fry zucchinis in a large pan by extra virgin olive oil over low heat or microwave it. For more crispiness, you may need to broil fried zucchinis.

UC-related Tips:

- Do not use garlic powder if you cannot tolerate it or if you have a flare-up.

Nutrition Facts

Servings: 2

Amount per serving

Calories	95
	% Daily Value*
Total Fat 7.4g	10%
Saturated Fat 1.1g	5%
Cholesterol 0mg	0%
Sodium 20mg	1%
Total Carbohydrate 7.2g	3%
Dietary Fiber 2.3g	8%
Total Sugars 3.6g	
Protein 2.8g	
Vitamin D 0mcg	0%
Calcium 32mg	2%
Iron 1mg	5%
Potassium 528mg	11%

HEALTHY POTATO CHIPS

Crunchy and healthy potato chips can be a tasty snack for Ulcerative Colitis patients as they can be made with no oil, and as the snack is fat-free.

- Prep Time: 10 minutes
- Cook Time: 10 minutes
- Total Time: 20 minutes
- Serving: 2

Ingredients

- 2 medium potatoes, skin removed
- ½ teaspoon garlic powder (optional)

- ½ teaspoon onion powder (optional)
- Salt, to taste

Instructions

1. Wash potatoes and then, peel-off the skins.
2. Slice potatoes into chips using a very thin slicer.
3. Add salt, garlic powder (optional), and onion powder (optional).
4. Spread all chips on a parchment paper sheet.
5. Put in the microwave until golden brown. Enjoy!

Cooking Tips:

- Potato chips perfectly match with any avocado snack.

UC-related Tips:

- Do not use garlic or onion powder when you are experiencing a flare-up. Make chips with salt only.

Nutrition Facts

Servings: 2

Amount per serving	
Calories	**151**
	% Daily Value*
Total Fat 0.2g	0%
Saturated Fat 0.1g	0%
Cholesterol 0mg	0%
Sodium 13mg	1%
Total Carbohydrate 34.5g	13%
Dietary Fiber 5.2g	19%
Total Sugars 2.6g	
Protein 3.8g	
Vitamin D 0mcg	0%
Calcium 22mg	2%
Iron 1mg	6%
Potassium 890mg	19%

DRINKS

RECOMMENDED HOT BEVERAGES

Recommended hot beverages for Ulcerative Colitis patients are:

- <u>Decaffeinated coffee:</u> use decaffeinated coffee instead of caffeinated coffee if you are experiencing a flare-up. When you are in remission, make sure you are taking caffeinated drinks in moderation. It is recommended not to take caffeinated drinks at all if you can.
- <u>Decaffeinated black tea:</u> if you would like to have earl gray, English breakfast, or any types of black tea, it is better to drink decaffeinated kinds, especially if you are experiencing a flare-up. If you are in remission, take caffeinated black tea in moderation. As cinnamon has anti-inflammatory properties, it is a great idea to pour a little bit of cinnamon powder in your black tea.
- <u>Peppermint Tea:</u> this herbal tea is an excellent choice for Ulcerative Colitis patients as it has properties that can soothe your digestive tract inflammation. Studies show that peppermint oil can help spasms and cramping in patients with gastrointestinal issues.
- <u>Green Tea:</u> is another excellent choice for Ulcerative Colitis patients. It includes polyphenol antioxidants such as epigallocatechin gallate (EGCG), a type of catechin that protects cells from damages and can reduce inflammation that can help chronic conditions. It can also help inhibit bacterial growth, which lowers the risks of getting infections. Moreover, green tea contains less caffeine than regular coffee. However, it could give you a similar mood.
- <u>Ziziphora/Oregano/Thyme Tea:</u> This herbal tea is recommended for people with Ulcerative Colitis.

Ziziphora is the name of a mountain plant from the Lamiaceae group, similar to Thyme. It has flavonoids with anti-inflammatory properties. Oregano contains great antioxidants such as Carvacrol and Thymol that can reduce the risk of virus activities. Studies have shown excellent anti-inflammatory properties of oregano. Thyme tea is also great for people with UC. It has antioxidants and antimicrobial properties with valuable sources of Iron. Thyme can also be used in foods as a great seasoning. You can pour one tablespoon of Ziziphora or Oregano or Thyme in a cup of boiling water and enjoy drinking this fantastic tea after 8-10 minutes.

- <u>Turmeric and Ginger Tea:</u> both turmeric and ginger are fantastic for people living with UC. Turmeric and Ginger have been used widely in ancient medicine. They use turmeric and ginger as medicines and for better digestion. Turmeric is high in antioxidants that can protect your cells from damaging and reduces the risks of getting infections. Curcumin in turmeric is a great anti-inflammatory ingredient. Ginger also has strong anti-inflammatory properties that can help reduce inflammation in the GI tract.
    - For making a great tea, add ½ teaspoon of ground turmeric and ½ teaspoon of freshly grated ginger in 2 cups of boiling water and enjoy your drink after 12-15 minutes. You can add 1-teaspoon honey or maple syrup to your tea if you can tolerate it. On of the delicious hot beverages you can make with Turmeric and Ginger is called Golden Milk.
    - Golden Milk: mix ½ cup of unsweetened almond milk or lactose-free cow milk, one teaspoon turmeric, ½ teaspoon of freshly

grated ginger, ½ teaspoon of cinnamon powder, and one teaspoon of honey or maple syrup (optional: if you can tolerate) in a small pot and boil. After boiling, simmer for 5 minutes until flavors over low heat.

- Ginger-Mint Tea: you can benefit from both ginger and mint properties by making this great tea. Mint has menthol, which helps reduce inflammation in the gut.

  Boil 10-15 mint leaves with one tablespoon of lemon juice and ½ teaspoon of freshly grated ginger and 2 cups of water in a small pot. Remove from heat, wait for three more minutes and add one tablespoon honey or maple syrup (optional: if you can tolerate) for sweetness if you want.

- Slippery Elm Tea: recent studies showed that slippery elm bark could soothe the stomach and intestinal linings and reducing inflammation and is an excellent drink for people with UC. Pour one tablespoon of slippery elm in a cup of boiling water and enjoy drinking after 10 minutes.

- Calendula Tea: this tea is known for helping people with peptic ulcers, reflux, and IBD. It can soothe gut inflammation and irritation as it has anti-inflammatory and wound-healing properties. Pour 1 tablespoon of dried calendula in a cup of boiling water and enjoy drinking after 10-12 minutes.

- Milk?: Generally speaking, Ulcerative Colitis patients can use low-fat milk if they are in remission and not lactose-intolerant. You can serve milk, hot or cold.
  - Some researchers recommend not to use regular cow milk or any nut/wild rice milk

when you are in a flare-up as milk is hard to be digested.

- o If you are in remission and not lactose-intolerant, it is recommended to consume low-fat cow milk, unsweetened almond milk, or rice milk. You can also use soy milk during remissions, but make sure you are using a Non-GMO type. Always check your intolerance level.
- o Some patients are lactose-intolerant due to UC. These patients can use low-fat, lactose-free cow milk, unsweetened almond milk, Non-GMO soy milk, and/or rice milk when they are in remission.

RECOMMENDED COLD BEVERAGES

Recommended cold beverages for Ulcerative Colitis patients are as below:

- Water: The best drink for Ulcerative Colitis patients is water. Try drinking at least 8-10 glasses of water each day, especially if you are experiencing a flare-up, which helps reduce your inflammation and relieve your diarrhea. Try not to use carbonated water if you have UC.
  - o Some patients experienced better feelings of consuming alkaline water with 9.5 pH. Alkaline water is water with a pH of more than 7 (normal). As it has a higher pH than regular water, some claim that it can balance body pH level. Most soda drinks in the market have acidic properties (pH smaller than 7). Ionized alkaline water can increase hydration as ionization may reduce the size of

molecular clusters of water. Some experts also claimed that as active oxygen in water is a free radical, it might damage healthy tissues. Alkaline water may neutralize active oxygen and avoid those damaging healthy tissues.

- <u>Do not drink</u> soda, carbonated beverages, and caffeinated beverages if you have UC. These drinks may cause you diarrhea and bloating, which can be active or severe your symptoms.
- <u>Gatorade/Powerade:</u> is a fantastic electrolyte drink for Ulcerative Colitis patients if they are in remission. It can help to relieve diarrhea, and it contains useful minerals such as sodium, potassium, and vitamins such as B3, B6, and B12.
  - o When you are in flare-up periods, try your electrolyte recipe: First glass: mix one cup of water with ½ teaspoon of sugar or honey and a pinch of salt. Second glass: mix one cup of boiled water with ¼ teaspoon of baking soda. When in hydration, drink half of the first glass and then half of the second glass. Drink more from glasses, respectively, if you are still thirsty.
- <u>Fruit Juices:</u> Fruit juices are excellent sources of vitamins for Ulcerative Colitis patients. Juicing is essential for Ulcerative Colitis patients, as many of them cannot digest fibers in foods and fruits easily. Hence, they can boost their nutrient intake by juicing. However, people with UC need to consume specific fruits with specific instructions:
  - o Do not use juices with the pulp.

- It is recommended not to add sugar or any artificial sweeteners to juices. If you can tolerate honey, maple syrup, or stevia, you can add them to your juice.
- Make sure peeling off fruit skins when you are juicing them.
- It is recommended to consume peeled and poached fruits/ fruit juices when you are experiencing a severe flare-up.
- The best fruit juice that can be consumed in moderation by Ulcerative Colitis patients are: Aloe Vera, Papaya, Honeydew Melon, Banana, Carrot, Cantaloupe, Pineapples, Squash, Pumpkin, Cucumber (peeled)
- You may want to try other fruit juices (skin removed) such as apple, peach, mango or pear when you are in remission. You may also juice vegetables such as celery and spinach during your remission period. Always start consuming less and check your tolerance level.
- Many experts recommend not to use fruits with small seeds such as blueberries and strawberries.
- Many Ulcerative Colitis patients can't tolerate tomato juice. Try not to consume it, especially if you are in a flare-up.

It is better to purchase organic fruits and always correctly wash fruits first, even if you know that you want to remove their skin.

Chapter 6. Food Preparation & Meal Planning for Ulcerative Colitis patients

The following tips can help you to have an effective food preparation and meal planning:

Eating Habits

1- Eat smaller portions, but frequent meals 5 to 6 times a day.
2- Keep yourself hydrated. Drink plenty of water and other allowed juices during a day. Pump-up your electrolyte intake, especially during flares using low-sugar sports drinks or use yours at home.
3- Drink slowly and chew well.
4- Do not use straw as you may ingest air, which can cause producing gas.
5- You can drink recommended herbal teas after your meal for better digestion, especially if you think that you ate a lot of your meal was heavy for you.
6- Give time to your herbal tea to brew well.
7- Eat your meal in peace and comfort in a relaxed place. Do not talk too much when you are eating your meal.
8- Do not work with your phone or laptop while eating your meals.
9- Do not drink water in the middle of eating meals.
10- Do not skip your breakfast at all.
11- Do not starve yourself. Determine correct specific times for your meals and stick to those times.
12- Do not eat very late. Eat dinner at least 2 hours before your sleep time, or 3 to 4 hours after your lunch.

13- Always have a meal plan and follow it. The worst thing for you is not knowing what to eat and what to cook.

14- Reduce consuming alcohol, sugar, and caffeinated drink during remission. Avoid consuming them in flare-up periods.

15- Do not leave your foods at normal temperature for more than 2 hours.

GROCERY SHOPPING

1- To prepare your meals in advance, you need to create a list before you go to the supermarket for daily or weekly shopping.

2- The list should include ingredients you need for your daily or weekly cooking plan. Remember that the ingredients should be well-tolerated.

3- Always try to purchase organic, non-GMO ingredients

4- Always try to buy lower-fat options.

5- For eggs, try to purchase organic, free-range types

6- For meat or pork, try to pick low-fat lean cuts

7- For poultry, skin-removed breasts and legs are the best options.

8- For cheese, try to purchase low-fat options. If you are lactose-intolerant, choose lactose-free cheese options. Use cheese in moderation only during the remission period.

9- For milk, try to purchase low-fat options. If you are lactose-intolerant, choose lactose-free milk options such as almond milk or rice milk. Use milk in moderation only during the remission period.

10- For grains, try not to get whole-wheat or whole-grain options.

11- For bread, try to find white bread that is not highly processed. For instance, pita bread might be a good option.

12- For baking, purchase all-purpose white flour. If you are gluten intolerant, use gluten-free options such as almond flour.

13- Purchase ripe bananas to test your tolerance. Use banana regularly if you can tolerate it.

14- For oil, purchase extra virgin olive oil or avocado oil.

15- Keep having turmeric, ginger, and cinnamon in your kitchen cabinet.

16- Avoid purchasing processed foods.

17- For sauces such as mayonnaise, try to purchase organic low fat and low sodium types.

18- For beef, chicken, or vegetable broth, try to buy organic low sodium types.

19- Always purchase organic potatoes.

20- It is not recommended to purchase fruit juices with pulp, added sugar, and juices from concentrate.

21- If you want to purchase almond butter, get the organic and smooth one.

22- Purchase stevia as a plant-based sweetener instead of refined sugars.

23- Try to purchase fresh foods instead of frozen or canned foods.

24- Read the ingredients of the snack you may want to purchase. Make sure that you can tolerate ingredients well.

25- Remember to have excellent foods such as papaya, butter lettuce, and cantaloupe in your basket.

COOKING TOOLS

You do not necessarily need to buy any specific tools to cook for an Ulcerative Colitis patient, but here are some of the tools that can help you ease the cooking process:

1- Cast Iron skillet: some people suggest having an iron skillet to absorb iron better, which may help Ulcerative Colitis patients with malabsorption to absorb the iron better.

2- Blender: for those who can use nuts in moderation, they need to blend them well. Having a suitable blender/mixer can help you cook well-blended meals such as soups, smoothies, nut butter, and juices.

3- Juicer: having a powerful juicer can help you taking the juices of fruits and vegetables without taking their fibers. With this tool, you may have fruits or vegetables that cannot be tolerated because of having high insoluble fiber.

4- Small lunch-dinner boxes: it is recommended for Ulcerative Colitis patients to eat smaller portions six times a day. One great idea to follow this eating style is to provide lunch, snacks, and dinners in separate boxes. For instance, you can put your lunch in two small lunch boxes instead of a big one and eat each box separately (e.g., with two hours of time-difference) at your workplace.

5- Spiralizer: to have spaghetti-like zucchini, potatoes, and squash, you may need to have a spiralizer.

6- Air fryer: air frying can be a great cooking option, as it does not need much oil. You can make great zucchini or potato chip snacks or other meals using an air fryer.

7- Timer and thermometer: both are helpful tools for you to cook delicious meals. Remember that meats should be cooked well for Ulcerative Colitis patients.

Hence, you can use these tools to check if inside meats cooked well or not.

KITCHEN PREPARATION

Here are some of the tips to prepare the kitchen before cooking:

1. Wash your hands perfectly when you want to cook.
2. Always wash fruits and vegetables before using them.
3. Remember to use allowed skin-removed or poached fruits.
4. Remember not to consume fruit cores or vegetable seeds.
5. Wash meats before cooking. Use disposable gloves when washing meats and put gloves in the garbage after. Always wash your hands with warm water right after washing meats and poultries.
6. Use a separate cutting board for raw meat
7. Keep raw meats away from other foods in the kitchen and fridge.
8. Never mix cooked foods with raw meats. Mixing can happen in plates, cutting boards, etc. Never eat such foods.
9. Remember to cook or boil meats, seafood, and vegetables in perfection.
10. Keep the kitchen area well-cleaned and sanitized.

MEAL PLANNING

1- Use proper cooking methods explained in this book. Keep your cooking style simple:

a. If you are in remission, you are free to apply cooking techniques such as stir-fry foods in moderation with extra virgin olive oil.

b. If you are in a flare, try to stick to techniques such as boiling, steaming, and poaching.

c. Grating spices such as ginger is better than consuming not-fresh powders.

2- You should have your meal plans ready for both remission and flare-up periods. Use the information on this book to create your meal plans for both mentioned periods. The plans should include:

a. Foods to avoid/to consume during a flare-up period

b. Foods to avoid/to consume during a remission period

3- You also should know the strategy of finding triggering foods for yourself. To keep it simple, if you ate a specific food at any time and observed any symptoms such as diarrhea, cramping, gas, bloating, and abdominal pain, you might be intolerant to that particular food. If you ate a meal and you are not sure about the ingredient(s) you are intolerant inside, you have to write this meal in your journal and record your symptoms and conditions there. Then, you need to review your journal at the end of each week or two again and check if you can find any relations or common ingredient(s) between different meals you could not tolerate or not. You can visit a dietitian or a nutritionist to guide you more on how to find triggering foods.

4- Create at least two, two-week meal plans for both periods (remission and flare), with enough variety and stick to them according to your health condition.

Your meal plan should have the following cooking/eating items:

    a. Meal-1: Breakfast
    b. Meal-2: Snack
    c. Meal-3: Lunch-1
    d. Meal-4: Lunch-2
    e. Meal-5: Snack
    f. Meal-6: Dinner
    g. Eight glasses of drinks

Soup, salad, appetizer, and dessert options should be added to your schedules as well. The next chapter of this book presents two detailed examples of biweekly meal plans. After the examples, this book gives you two blank meal plans. You can fill the blanked spaces to design your two-week meal plan.

5- If you are working outside the home, plan to cook for your next day's lunch at work.

6- Prepare or purchase a journal designed explicitly for Ulcerative Colitis patients to keep the records of your meals taken and symptoms you may experience.

OTHER TIPS

1- As an advanced technique, you can prepare different meal plans for different seasons, which can help you use fresh seasonal ingredients in your meals.

2- This book helps you cooking fast and easy delicious meals for Ulcerative Colitis patients. However, allocate time as much as you can for your cooking.

    a. Presentation is very important to increase the appetite. If you see cooking as an art, you can definitely prepare meals with an excellent presentation based on your artistic and creative ideas.

b. Try to have colorful meals that can increase your appetite, as well. Have your main course with colorful sides such as green (zucchinis), orange (carrots), yellow (lemon wedges or potatoes), etc.

c. Be creative: by reading this book and your hard work on finding the best tolerable foods, you now know which ingredients are great, which are safe and which are okay during remission. Now, you can create your meals or judge any meal recipe based on your knowledge.

3- Using alkaline water: there are not many scientific studies about the impact of using alkaline waters on Ulcerative Colitis patients. However, some patients found that the alkaline water (known as Kangen water in some references) could reduce their symptoms, and they had longer remission periods. Other properties of alkaline-water machines might also be helpful. For example, alkaline water machines typically produce waters with low pH (e.g., 2.5 pH) that possibly remove pesticides from the skin of foods such as fruits, vegetables, and rice (if you wash them with such waters). Hence, consuming alkaline water might be an option to investigate for you.

CHAPTER 7. BI-WEEKLY COOKING PLAN FOR ULCERATIVE COLITIS PATIENTS

This chapter provides you with an example of a biweekly meal plan for remission periods. It can give you an idea of how to create your biweekly plans for remission and flare-up periods.

Here are some of the essential tips you need to remember when you want to make your meal plan for remission periods:

COOKING PLAN FOR REMISSION PERIODS:

-   Try varieties of foods, but always eat and drink healthy foods.
-   If you are lactose-intolerant, try alternative products explained in this book.
-   If you are gluten-intolerant, try alternative products explained in this book.
-   When you are in remission, it does not mean that you can eat everything. There are still some triggering foods to avoid as they can wake up flares. Always make your meal plan based on your health conditions and non-triggering foods that can be well-tolerated by you.
-   If you are sensitive to seafood, you can substitute seafood with other foods with healthy fat and protein sources. Many non-seafood cooking recipes provided for you in this book.
-   Remember that it is recommended to eat six portions a day instead of 3 portions. Hence, you can have breakfast, snack (between breakfast and lunch),

lunch, snack (between lunch and dinner), dinner, and snack (between dinner and your sleep time). You can use appetizers, snacks, desserts, and snack recipes in this book for snack portions. Alternatively, you can have soups or salads as before-lunch or before-dinner snacks.

Here is an example of a biweekly meal plan for remission Periods:

Week-1:	Week-2:
Monday	Monday
Breakfast: Avocado Egg Breakfast Toast	**Breakfast:** Egg Tacos with Avocado
Snack-1: Zucchini Chips	**Snack-1:** Gluten-Free Rice Crackers
Lunch: Chicken Kebab (From Last Night)	**Lunch:** Chicken Stroganoff (From Last Night)
Snack-2: Banana Milkshake	**Snack-2:** Cooler Drink or Almond Butter Toast
Dinner: Grilled Honey Salmon and/or Carrot Potato Soup	**Dinner:** Lemon Steamed Halibut with White Rice
Snack-3: Diced Fruits	**Snack-3:** Apple Ginger Sundae
Drinks: Coffee, Peppermint Tea	**Drinks:** Earl Gray Tea, Green Tea
Tuesday	Tuesday
Breakfast: Almond Butter Banana Sandwich	**Breakfast:** Fruit Salad with Almond Milk
Snack-1: Gluten-Free Ginger Biscuit	**Snack-1:** Avocado Dip
Lunch: Grilled Honey Salmon and/or Carrot Potato Soup	**Lunch:** Lemon Steamed Halibut with White Rice
Snack-2: Avocado Smoothie	**Snack-2:** Banana Cinnamon Smoothie
Dinner: Potato Cutlet with Stracciatella Soup	**Dinner:** Classic Tuna Pasta Salad or Butternut Squash Soup
Snack-3: Applesauce	**Snack-3:** Pomegranate Angelica Drink
Drinks: Decaffeinated Black Tea, Green Tea	**Drinks:** Decaffeinated Coffee, Peppermint Tea
Wednesday	Wednesday
Breakfast: Apple Cinnamon Oatmeal	**Breakfast:** Pineapple Ginger Oatmeal
Snack-1: Tofu Toast	**Snack-1:** Guacamole-Like Snack
Lunch: Potato Cutlet with Stracciatella Soup	**Lunch:** Classic Tuna Pasta Salad or Butternut Squash Soup
Snack-2: Cantaloupe Smoothie	**Snack-2:** Banana Milkshake
Dinner: Balsamic Peach Pork	**Dinner:** Olivier/Potato Salad with Pumpkin Soup
Snack-3: Poached Fruit Compote	**Snack-3:** Cantaloupe Mix Smoothie
Drinks: Decaffeinated Coffee, Peppermint Tea	**Drinks:** Coffee, Oregano Tea
Thursday	Thursday
Breakfast: Gluten-Free Fluffy Pancakes	**Breakfast:** Baked Apple
Snack-1: Cheese Sticks	**Snack-1:** Avocado Cheese Bagel
Lunch: Balsamic Peach Pork	**Lunch:** Olivier/Potato Salad with Pumpkin Soup
Snack-2: Peach Mango Banana Smoothie	**Snack-2:** Baba Ghanoush
Dinner: Thunfisch Pizza and/or Butternut Squash Soup	**Dinner:** Grilled Beef Kebab with White Rice
Snack-3: Gluten-Free Apple Pie	**Snack-3:** Carrot Juice with Mango Ice Cream
Drinks: Black Tea with Cinnamon, Ginger Mint Tea	**Drinks:** Decaffeinated Earl Grey Tea, Ginger Mint Tea
Friday	Friday
Breakfast: Two Poached Eggs with Toasts	**Breakfast:** Almond Butter Honey Banana Toast
Snack-1: Almond Butter Sandwich	**Snack-1:** Applesauce
Lunch: Thunfisch Pizza and/or Butternut Squash Soup	**Lunch:** Grilled Beef Kebab with White Rice
Snack-2: Banana Cinnamon Smoothie	**Snack-2:** Carrot Avocado Salad

Dinner: Chicken Zucchini Stew with Chicken Broth **Snack-3:** Diced Fruits such as Papaya **Drinks:** Decaffeinated Coffee, Ziziphora Tea	**Dinner:** Chicken Pineapple Pizza **Snack-3:** Warm Apple Crumble **Drinks:** Decaffeinated Coffee, Green Tea
Saturday	Saturday
Breakfast: Avocado Cheese Bagel **Snack-1:** Poached Fruits with Plain Yogurt **Lunch:** Chicken Zucchini Stew with Chicken Broth **Snack-2:** Butter Lettuce Salad **Dinner:** Hungarian Goulash with Bone Broth **Snack-3:** Lemon Sorbet or a Fruit Juice **Drinks:** Coffee, Turmeric Ginger Tea	**Breakfast:** Egg Salmon Avocado **Snack-1:** Tofu Toast **Lunch:** Chicken Pineapple Pizza **Snack-2:** Applesauce Avocado Smoothie **Dinner:** Chicken & Shrimp Teriyaki with Rice Noodles **Snack-3:** Rice Pudding **Drinks:** Coffee, Turmeric Ginger Tea
Sunday	Sunday
Breakfast: Smoothie Bowl with Almond Milk **Snack-1:** Gluten-Free Rice Crackers **Lunch:** Hungarian Goulash with Bone Broth **Snack-2:** Hummus **Dinner:** Chicken Stroganoff **Snack-3:** Avocado Peach Popsicle **Drinks:** Decaffeinated Coffee, Slippery Elm Tea	**Breakfast:** Zucchini Bread Oatmeal **Snack-1:** Gluten-Free Ginger Biscuit **Lunch:** Chicken & Shrimp Teriyaki with Rice Noodles **Snack-2:** Apple Pear Salad **Dinner:** Ginger Sticky Pork **Snack-3:** Pineapple Cake Sundae **Drinks:** Decaffeinated Black Tea, Calendula Tea

Here are some of the critical points you need to remember when you want to make your meal plan for flare-up periods:

COOKING PLAN FOR FLARE-UP PERIODS

- You have to limit yourself to non-triggering healthy food recipes.
- It is recommended to avoid consuming lactose and gluten during flares.
- Remember: when you are in a flare, you have to put more non-triggering soups, juices, and broth in your meal plan.
- Always make your meal plan based on your health conditions and non-triggering foods that can be well-tolerated by you.

- During flares, stick to your meal plan and modify it only if you found any intolerable foods/ingredients.
- Put more foods with anti-inflammatory herbs and spices such as turmeric and ginger in your flare-up meal plan.
- Drink safe anti-inflammatory herbal teas such as peppermint and green tea during flare-up periods.
- If you are sensitive to seafood, you can substitute seafood with other foods with healthy fat and protein sources. Many non-seafood cooking recipes provided for you in this book.
- Remember that it is recommended to eat six portions a day instead of three portions. Hence, you can have breakfast, snack (between breakfast and lunch), lunch, snack (between lunch and dinner), dinner, and snack (between dinner and your sleep time). You can use appetizers, snacks, desserts, and snack recipes in this book for snack portions. Alternatively, you can have soups or salads as before-lunch or before-dinner snacks.
- If you have issues in making an effective meal plan for your flare-up periods, ask support from a nutritionist or a dietitian. Here is an example of a biweekly flare-up meal plan:

Week-1:	Week-2:
Monday	**Monday**
Breakfast: Avocado + 2 Poached Eggs **Snack-1:** Zucchini Salad **Lunch:** Chicken Kebab with White Rice (From Last Night) **Snack-2:** Carrot Juice **Dinner:** Boiled Salmon / Carrot Potato Soup **Snack-3:** Diced Non-Triggering Fruits **Drinks:** Decaffeinated Coffee, Peppermint Tea	**Breakfast:** Two Poached Eggs with Avocado **Snack-1:** Avocado Dip **Lunch:** Chicken Noodle Soup (From Last Night) **Snack-2:** Cooler Drink **Dinner:** Lemon Steamed Halibut with White Rice **Snack-3:** Ginger Fruit Sherbet (Sweetened by Stevia) **Drinks:** Decaffeinated Black Tea, Green Tea
Tuesday	**Tuesday**
Breakfast: Smooth Almond Butter Banana Sandwich **Snack-1:** Gluten-Free Ginger Biscuit or Rice Crackers **Lunch:** Boiled Salmon / Carrot Potato Soup **Snack-2:** Cantaloupe Juice **Dinner:** Turkey Pot Pie Soup **Snack-3:** Applesauce **Drinks:** Decaffeinated Black Tea, Green Tea	**Breakfast:** Fruit Salad **Snack-1:** Oatmeal (if tolerable) or Firm Tofu **Lunch:** Lemon Steamed Halibut with White Rice **Snack-2:** Carrot Juice **Dinner:** Classic Tuna Pasta Salad + One Bone Broth Cup **Snack-3:** Pomegranate Angelica Drink **Drinks:** Decaffeinated Coffee, Peppermint Tea
Wednesday	**Wednesday**
Breakfast: Oatmeal (if tolerable) or Safe Fruit Bowl **Snack-1:** Firm Tofu Toast **Lunch:** Turkey Pot Pie Soup **Snack-2:** Honeydew Melon Juice **Dinner:** Bone Broth + Carrot Avocado Salad **Snack-3:** Poached Fruit Compote (e.g., Peeled Apple) **Drinks:** Green Tea, Peppermint Tea	**Breakfast:** Oatmeal (if tolerable) or a Safe Fruit Bowl **Snack-1:** Guacamole-Like Snack **Lunch:** Classic Tuna Pasta Salad + One Bone Broth Cup **Snack-2:** Diced Banana **Dinner:** Potato Salad + Pumpkin Soup **Snack-3:** Cantaloupe Juice **Drinks:** Green Tea, Peppermint Tea
Thursday	**Thursday**
Breakfast: Two Poached Eggs with Toasts **Snack-1:** Diced Fruits **Lunch:** Bone Broth + Carrot Avocado Salad **Snack-2:** Applesauce Avocado Smoothie (Lactose-Free) **Dinner:** Butternut Squash Soup **Snack-3:** Cantaloupe or Watermelon Juice **Drinks:** Decaffeinated Black Tea, Ginger Mint Tea	**Breakfast:** Baked Apple **Snack-1:** Smooth Almond Butter Sandwich **Lunch:** Potato Salad + Pumpkin Soup **Snack-2:** Poached Egg Avocado White Pita **Dinner:** Turkey Zucchini Noodles **Snack-3:** Carrot Juice **Drinks:** Decaffeinated Earl Grey Tea, Ginger Mint Tea
Friday	**Friday**

Breakfast: Avocado + Gluten-Free Bagel **Snack-1:** Almond Butter Sandwich **Lunch:** Butternut Squash Soup **Snack-2:** Applesauce **Dinner:** Chicken Zucchini Stew with Chicken Broth **Snack-3:** Diced Fruits such as Papaya **Drinks:** Decaffeinated Coffee, Peppermint Tea	**Breakfast:** Almond Butter Honey Banana Toast **Snack-1:** Applesauce **Lunch:** Turkey Zucchini Noodles **Snack-2:** Carrot Avocado Salad **Dinner:** Butternut Squash Soup **Snack-3:** Lemon Sorbet **Drinks:** Peppermint Tea, Green Tea
Saturday	Saturday
Breakfast: Smooth Almond Butter Banana Sandwich **Snack-1:** Poached Fruits (Unsweetened or with Stevia) **Lunch:** Chicken Zucchini Stew with Chicken Broth **Snack-2:** Ginger Cool Drink **Dinner:** Bone Broth and Mashed Potato with No Milk **Snack-3:** Lemon Sorbet **Drinks:** Turmeric Ginger Tea, Turmeric Ginger Tea	**Breakfast:** 2 Poached Eggs with Avocado **Snack-1:** Firm Tofu Toast **Lunch:** Butternut Squash Soup **Snack-2:** Papaya Dices **Dinner:** Lemon Shrimp with White Rice **Snack-3:** Rice Pudding (Unsweetened or by Stevia) **Drinks:** Decaffeinated Coffee, Turmeric Ginger Tea
Sunday	Sunday
Breakfast: Smoothie Bowl with Almond Milk **Snack-1:** Gluten-Free Rice Crackers or Applesauce **Lunch:** Bone Broth and Mashed Potato with No Milk **Snack-2:** Guacamole Like Snack **Dinner:** Chicken Noodle Soup **Snack-3:** Popsicle from a Non-triggering Fruit **Drinks:** Decaffeinated Coffee, Green Tea	**Breakfast:** Zucchini Bread Oatmeal **Snack-1:** Gluten-Free Ginger Biscuit **Lunch:** Lemon Shrimp with White Rice **Snack-2:** Apple Pear Salad **Dinner:** Stracciatella Soup + Zucchini Salad **Snack-3:** Popsicle from a Non-triggering Fruit **Drinks:** Decaffeinated Black Tea, Peppermint Tea

BIWEEKLY COOKING PLAN FOR ULCERATIVE COLITIS PATIENTS – BLANK

This section gives you two free blank meal plan tables that can be filled by you if you want to create your biweekly plans for remission and flare-up periods.

Biweekly Meal Plan for Remission Periods	
Week-1:	Week-2:
Monday	Monday
Breakfast: Snack-1: Lunch: Snack-2: Dinner: Snack-3: Drinks:	Breakfast: Snack-1: Lunch: Snack-2: Dinner: Snack-3: Drinks:
Tuesday	Tuesday
Breakfast: Snack-1: Lunch: Snack-2: Dinner: Snack-3: Drinks:	Breakfast: Snack-1: Lunch: Snack-2: Dinner: Snack-3: Drinks:
Wednesday	Wednesday
Breakfast: Snack-1: Lunch: Snack-2: Dinner: Snack-3: Drinks:	Breakfast: Snack-1: Lunch: Snack-2: Dinner: Snack-3: Drinks:
Thursday	Thursday
Breakfast: Snack-1: Lunch: Snack-2: Dinner: Snack-3: Drinks:	Breakfast: Snack-1: Lunch: Snack-2: Dinner: Snack-3: Drinks:
Friday	Friday
Breakfast: Snack-1: Lunch: Snack-2: Dinner: Snack-3: Drinks:	Breakfast: Snack-1: Lunch: Snack-2: Dinner: Snack-3: Drinks:
Saturday	Saturday
Breakfast: Snack-1: Lunch: Snack-2: Dinner: Snack-3: Drinks:	Breakfast: Snack-1: Lunch: Snack-2: Dinner: Snack-3: Drinks:
Sunday	Sunday
Breakfast: Snack-1: Lunch: Snack-2: Dinner: Snack-3: Drinks:	Breakfast: Snack-1: Lunch: Snack-2: Dinner: Snack-3: Drinks:

Biweekly Meal Plan for Flare-Up Periods	
Week-1:	**Week-2:**
Monday	Monday
Breakfast: Snack-1: Lunch: Snack-2: Dinner: Snack-3: Drinks:	Breakfast: Snack-1: Lunch: Snack-2: Dinner: Snack-3: Drinks:
Tuesday	Tuesday
Breakfast: Snack-1: Lunch: Snack-2: Dinner: Snack-3: Drinks:	Breakfast: Snack-1: Lunch: Snack-2: Dinner: Snack-3: Drinks:
Wednesday	Wednesday
Breakfast: Snack-1: Lunch: Snack-2: Dinner: Snack-3: Drinks:	Breakfast: Snack-1: Lunch: Snack-2: Dinner: Snack-3: Drinks:
Thursday	Thursday
Breakfast: Snack-1: Lunch: Snack-2: Dinner: Snack-3: Drinks:	Breakfast: Snack-1: Lunch: Snack-2: Dinner: Snack-3: Drinks:
Friday	Friday
Breakfast: Snack-1: Lunch: Snack-2: Dinner: Snack-3: Drinks:	Breakfast: Snack-1: Lunch: Snack-2: Dinner: Snack-3: Drinks:
Saturday	Saturday
Breakfast: Snack-1: Lunch: Snack-2: Dinner: Snack-3: Drinks:	Breakfast: Snack-1: Lunch: Snack-2: Dinner: Snack-3: Drinks:
Sunday	Sunday
Breakfast: Snack-1: Lunch: Snack-2: Dinner: Snack-3: Drinks:	Breakfast: Snack-1: Lunch: Snack-2: Dinner: Snack-3: Drinks:

CHAPTER 8. TOP 200 ULCERATIVE COLITIS TIPS & EATING PATTERNS

This chapter provides you with the top 200 tips and eating patterns an Ulcerative Colitis patient should follow. These tips summarize some of the essential tips in terms of UC lifestyle, diet, cooking recipes, cooking management, and meal planning this book enumerated in previous chapters. You may want to print these tips and have it with you to review. If you want to have high quality images, you can get the paperback version of this book available in amazon store.

1. *The Ulcerative Colitis Patients may have experience different symptoms and treatment plans compared with the Crohn's patients. Remember not to compare Ulcerative Colitis symptoms, management, and treatments with Crohn's symptoms, management, and treatment procedures, but increase your knowledge about different IBD symptoms. Some patients who have been diagnosed with Ulcerative Colitis might have Crohn's disease. Hence, learn about Crohn's symptoms and, if suspicious of any newly raised symptoms, visit your doctor as soon as possible.*
2. *Relax by doing 15-minutes meditation or yoga every day.*
3. *Try to follow your treatment procedure perfectly.*
4. *Have Ulcerative Colitis-friendly cooking plans.*
5. *Check possible governmental or insurance supports for your Ulcerative Colitis medications or medical procedures.*
6. *Create diet plans for flare and remission periods.*
7. *Record the history of your consumed foods & your symptoms in a journal for Ulcerative Colitis patients.*
8. *Eating slow, chew more.*
9. *Keep your Ulcerative Colitis knowledge updated.*
10. *Always remember: You are unique, and so do your Ulcerative Colitis conditions.*

11. *Do not be shy, talking about your Ulcerative Colitis conditions and feelings.*
12. *Visit your doctor as soon as possible if you experienced a new symptom or side effect.*
13. *Stay strong, be patient, and hopeful during flare-up periods.*
14. *Have bathroom request card/letter, wet wipes, small toilette paper, little sanitizer, tissue, small mirror, talcum powder, clean underwear, skin cream, freezer bag, and odor in your Emergency Kit.*
15. *Avoid drinking alcohol in flares. Drink moderately during Remissions.*
16. *If you want to tell a friend about your Ulcerative Colitis: Plan talking points in advance, find the right time to talk, explain conditions in the simplest way, explain your feelings during flares, explain how valuable your relationship is to you, and tell how she/he can be of any bit of help.*
17. *Do the Washroom Planning in advance: Ask then sit in restaurants!*
18. *If you want to get married, talk to your doctor about your decision.*
19. *For workplace management: Request bathroom breaks, talk to your boss & colleagues about your needs, have an emergency kit with you, have a desk closer to the washroom, ask if you can have flexible hours, and follow your workplace rights.*
20. *During pregnancy: Eat and drink healthy, non-triggering, and enough, take your medications and supplements as prescribed, monitor your pregnancy with doctors well.*
21. *If you want to get pregnant: Check your health condition with your doctor, make sure you are in remission for pregnancy, and talk to your doctor about medications and supplements you need to take.*
22. *After pregnancy tips: Delivery during remissions is close to the standard rate, eat and drink healthily during the*

breastfeeding period, and check your doctor to have safe medications during the breastfeeding period.

23. Do not skip a medication dose or a doctor's appointment. Always carefully follow your treatment plan.
24. Do not sleep late. Stick to your sleeping schedule.
25. Eat Small Portions 6 Times a Day.
26. If you think you will have stress during a medical procedure, ask support from a family member or a friend.
27. If you tried a lot but still have a problem making a strategic diet plan, seek help from a dietician.
28. If you feel depressed, visit a Psychologist.
29. Do not change your diet a lot. Have a strategic diet plan & improve it step by step.
30. Do not stay alone, especially on Saturday nights! Plan Saturday night outs in advance & remain social.
31. The best fertility time for Ulcerative Colitis patients: In remission periods. The fertility rate decreases in flare-up periods.
32. If you are unhappy with your relationship due to your Ulcerative Colitis conditions: Be frank about your condition, talk to your loved one about your feelings, ask support from psychologists, and stay positive.
33. Joining Ulcerative Colitis communities: Can keep you updated, can get support from other patients. You can participate in social activities, and you can help others as well.
34. Do not take NSAIDS without your doctor's permission.
35. Do not get dehydrated! Always have a bottle of water with you.
36. Do not think that you are cured as you are in remission! Continue the follow-up/check-up tests and procedures.
37. Do not use Antibiotics without your doctor's permission. Ask your doctor about the best treatment for you.
38. Always carefully wash fruits and vegetables before consuming them.

39. *Record your doctor appointments. Meet your doctor on a regular basis.*
40. *If you do not project a remission period soon, be patient. What comes up goes down!*
41. *Immunize yourself & record your immunization history.*
42. *Avoid overthinking! Ask your doctor's opinion.*
43. *Discuss with your doctor any natural products, supplements, or herbs you want to consume for your Ulcerative Colitis.*
44. *Do not forget to follow hygiene practices carefully.*
45. *Always care about prescribed supplements. Never miss any of your supplement doses.*
46. *It is recommended to avoid consuming lactose and gluten during flares.*
47. *When you are in remission, it does not mean that you can eat everything. There are still some triggering foods to avoid as they can wake up flares.*
48. *When you are in a flare, you have to put more non-triggering soups, juices, and broth in your meal plan.*
49. *Avoid high fiber foods during flare-up periods.*
50. *Put more foods with anti-inflammatory herbs and spices such as turmeric and ginger in your flare-up meal plan.*
51. *Drink safe anti-inflammatory herbal teas such as peppermint and green tea during flare-up periods.*
52. *Have an iron skillet to absorb iron better, which may help Ulcerative Colitis patients with malabsorption.*
53. *Never mix cooked foods with raw meats. Mixing can happen in plates, cutting boards, etc. Never eat such foods.*
54. *If you are in a flare, try to stick to techniques such as boiling, steaming, and poaching.*
55. *Create at least two, two-week meal plans for both periods (remission and flare), with enough variety and stick to them according to your health condition.*
56. *If you are working outside the home, plan to cook for your next day's lunch at work.*

57. To prepare your meals in advance, you need to create a list before you go to the supermarket for daily or weekly shopping.

58. Your shopping list should include ingredients you need for your daily or weekly cooking plan. Remember that the ingredients should be well-tolerated.

59. Always try to purchase organic, non-GMO ingredients

60. Always try to buy lower-fat options.

61. For eggs, try to purchase organic, free-range types.

62. For meat or pork, try to pick low-fat lean cuts.

63. For poultry, skin-removed breasts and legs are the best options.

64. For cheese, try to purchase low-fat options. If you are lactose-intolerant, choose lactose-free cheese options. Use cheese in moderation only during the remission period.

65. For milk, try to purchase low-fat options. If you are lactose-intolerant, choose lactose-free milk options such as almond milk or rice milk. Use milk in moderation only during the remission period.

66. For grains, try not to get whole-wheat or whole-grain options.

67. For bread, try to find white bread that is not highly processed. For instance, pita bread might be a good option.

68. For baking, purchase all-purpose white flour. If you are gluten intolerant, use gluten-free options such as almond flour.

69. For oil, purchase extra virgin olive oil or avocado oil.

70. Keep having turmeric, ginger, and cinnamon in your kitchen cabinet.

71. Avoid purchasing processed foods.

72. For sauces such as mayonnaise, try to purchase organic low fat and low sodium types and consume only during remissions.

73. For beef, chicken, or vegetable broth, try to buy organic low sodium types.

74. *Always purchase organic potatoes. White is preferred.*
75. *It is not recommended to purchase fruit juices with pulp, added sugar, and juices from concentrate.*
76. *If you want to purchase almond butter, get the organic and smooth one.*
77. *Purchase stevia as a plant-based sweetener instead of refined sugars.*
78. *Try to purchase fresh foods instead of frozen or canned foods.*
79. *Read the ingredients of the snack you may want to purchase. Make sure that you can tolerate all ingredients well.*
80. *Remember to have excellent foods such as papaya, butter lettuce, banana, and cantaloupe in your basket if you can tolerate them.*
81. *Put a variety of seafood in your biweekly meal plan if you are not allergic to them. Tuna, salmon, and shrimp are excellent sources of healthy fats and Omega-3.*
82. *If you want to consume non-triggering fruits during remission, remove their skins and cores.*
83. *The best way for Ulcerative Colitis patients to consume vegetables is to boil them.*
84. *Do not use straw as you may ingest air, which can cause producing gas.*
85. *You can drink recommended herbal teas after your meal for better digestion, especially if you think that you ate a lot of your meal was heavy for you. Give time to your herbal tea to brew well.*
86. *Eat your meal in peace and comfort in a relaxed place. Do not talk too much when you are eating your meal. Do not work with your phone or laptop while eating your meals.*
87. *Do not drink water in the middle of eating meals.*
88. *Do not skip your breakfast at all. High protein breakfast is an excellent option for Ulcerative Colitis patients.*
89. *Do not starve yourself. Determine correct specific times for your meals and stick to those times.*

90. Do not eat very late. Eat dinner at least 2 hours before your sleep time, or 3 to 4 hours after your lunch.

91. Always have a meal plan and follow it. The worst thing for you is not knowing what to eat and what to cook.

92. Reduce consuming sugar and caffeinated drink during remission. Avoid consuming them in flare-up periods.

93. Do not leave your foods at normal temperature for more than 2 hours.

94. Try drinking at least 8-10 glasses of water each day, especially if you are experiencing a flare-up, which helps reduce your inflammation and relieve your diarrhea.

95. Some patients experienced better feelings of consuming alkaline water with 9.5 pH. You may want to try the Alkaline water.

96. Do not drink soda, carbonated beverages, and caffeinated beverages if you have Ulcerative Colitis. These drinks may cause you diarrhea and bloating, which can be active or severe your symptoms.

97. Gatorade/Powerade: is a fantastic electrolyte drink for Ulcerative Colitis patients if they are in remission. It can help to relieve diarrhea, and it contains useful minerals such as sodium, potassium, and vitamins such as B3, B6, and B12. However, it is recommended to make your own electrolyte drink at home during flares.

98. The best fruit juice that can be consumed in moderation by Ulcerative Colitis patients are: Aloe Vera, Papaya, Honeydew Melon, Banana, Carrot, Cantaloupe, Pineapples, Squash, Pumpkin, Cucumber (peeled)

99. You may want to try other fruit juices (skin removed) such as apple, peach, mango or pear when you are in remission. You may also juice vegetables such as celery and spinach during your remission period. Always start consuming less and check your tolerance level.

100. Many experts recommend not using fruits with small seeds such as blueberries and strawberries.

101. Do not consume fried, greasy, and fatty foods, especially during flares.
102. Many Ulcerative Colitis patients cannot tolerate tomato. Try not to consume it in any form, especially if you are in a flare-up.
103. The best diet for an Ulcerative Colitis patient is her/his own created diet. The low residue and low fiber diets are helpful as well. Other diets, such as Paleo, Low-FODMAP, Microbiome, etc., have some excellent properties for Ulcerative Colitis patients. However, they are not as effective as they recommend some Ulcerative Colitis triggering foods.
104. Avoid Consuming Foods with High Saturated Trans Fat.
105. Some of the safe snacks can be Almond butter, oatmeal, applesauce, banana & homemade smoothies from non-triggering fruits.
106. Check your food tolerances during remissions. Consider possible further complications.
107. Try making pumpkin or squash Soups. Blend them during flares!
108. It is an excellent idea to putt bone, beef, chicken, or vegetable broths in your weekly meal plan.
109. Consume salt in moderation in your cooking.
110. Do not stick to the stir-frying method for cooking fishes. Try other methods such as boiling and grilling.
111. Always make sure inside meats cooked well.
112. Try Herbs such as Cumin, Bay leaves, Angelica & Thyme, & Oregano in Remissions
113. It is a good idea to use a proper Juicer to remove fiber from fruits & vegetables.
114. It is a good idea to use an air fryer for making delicious potato or zucchini chips.
115. Avoid cooking fatty parts of poultries, stick to Lean/Extra Lean parts of beef or pork.
116. It is essential to use a separate cutting board for raw meats.
117. Watch your sugar intake during remissions.

118. White rice & spaghetti squash are great alternatives for noodles.
119. Best sugar alternatives are stevia, honey, and maple syrup.
120. If you have both Ulcerative Colitis and IBS, avoid consuming FODMAP sugars.
121. Limit consuming sweet carbohydrates and added sugar products significantly.
122. It is not a bad idea to update your meal plan and cook seasonally.
123. If you cook for an Ulcerative Colitis patient, ask about food tolerances and non-triggering foods for cooking.
124. Butter tips: Use grass-fed butter in moderation during remission, and avoid using butter in flares.
125. Some of the lactose-free milk to consume are lactose-free cow milk, almond milk, rice milk, oat milk, and soy milk.
126. Some gluten-free flour alternatives: almond flour, oat flour & tapioca flour.
127. Best cooking methods during flares are boiling, poaching, steaming, stewing (using a little amount of safe oil), and baking (using a small amount of safe oil).
128. Best cooking methods during remissions are boiling, poaching, steaming, stewing, grilling, air frying, roasting, and baking.
129. Use safe proteins such as eggs and firm tofu.
130. Instead of potato fries, you can make skin-removed zucchini chips.
131. One of the best fruits with soluble fiber for Ulcerative Colitis patients is avocado!
132. Try not to smoke or vape or smoke moderately in remissions only.
133. Some of the great desserts for Ulcerative Colitis patients are popsicles and lactose-free sorbets from non-triggering fruits.
134. Avoid consuming nuts and seeds if you have any kind of narrowing or stricture complications.

135. Avoid consuming onion, garlic, and black pepper in flares. Use them in moderation during remission periods as well.
136. Do not consume spicy foods at all during flares. Try not to consume it during remissions as well.
137. The ostrich meat is an excellent option for Ulcerative Colitis patients. Choose the low-fat part if you want to cook it.
138. Try Butter lettuce if you want to make a garden salad. This type of lettuce can be more tolerated than other types of lettuce.
139. If you are suspicious about a fruit or a vegetable to consume, peel it, remove seeds/cores, boil it and then, eat it!
140. You can eat appetizers such as hummus in moderation during remissions.
141. Green peas might also be consumed during remission periods.
142. Put carrots in your meal plan as a great side dish choice.
143. Avoid eating chicken wings during flares & eat them moderately in remissions
144. The non-whole grain pasta is a great meal option for Ulcerative Colitis patients if they are not gluten-intolerant.
145. Banana can be tolerated well in most Ulcerative Colitis patients. Remember that ripe banana has less fiber, but more sugar and unripe banana has more fiber but less sugar. Try to check your tolerance regarding ripe and unripe bananas.
146. The best way to cook eggs is to boil them.
147. If you are lactose-intolerant, you can still consume cheese products during remissions. Make sure you are consuming lactose-free options. Some hard old-age cheeses are fine to consume as well.
148. Avoid consuming eggplants with lots of seeds during flares.
149. If you cannot tolerate mushrooms, try Shiitake mushrooms.
150. You can boil spinach and consume during flares. Always check your tolerance regarding spinach during flares and remissions.

151. Avoid eating high insoluble vegetables such as broccoli, cabbage, and cauliflower during flares. Check your tolerance during remissions as well.
152. If you want to eat cucumber, remove its skin first.
153. Avoid eating greasy and fatty sauces/gravies.
154. Going to the gym and have some proper exercises can help you keep your remission for a more extended period.
155. Reduce your stress level by doing exercises, meditation, yoga, and other relaxation techniques.
156. Avoid consuming jams or marmalades during flares.
157. Avoid consuming dried fruits, especially during flares.
158. Avoid consuming corn and popcorns during flares and remissions.
159. Avoid consuming pickles during flares. Consume pickles and sauerkraut in moderation during remissions.
160. Avoid consuming legumes during flares.
161. If you are a parent of a kid with Ulcerative Colitis, You need to be very patient with your kid. Treatment procedures could be very frustrating for them. Be with them on every step of the treatment.
162. If your loved one diagnosed with an Ulcerative Colitis, try to educate yourself, listen to your loved one, help them record their medical history, be with them during medical procedures, make proper cooking plans, give social life support, help her/him on the stress management, give physical supports, and be prepared for flare-up periods.
163. If planning any event, make sure a washroom is available nearby.
164. Before any travel, check the map and find washroom spots.
165. Schedule your social events according to your loved one's Ulcerative Colitis health condition. If she/he is in a flare-up period, it might not be an excellent time to celebrate! Do this for your special occasions if you can, as well.

166. If you plan to go to a restaurant, always check the menu to see if they have any food options match with your Ulcerative Colitis limitations.

167. If you are cooking for the next day lunch, a very great option is to prepare 2-3 small lunch boxes of food for them rather than a big lunch box to eat smaller portions.

168. Record any questions you want to ask your doctor in your Ulcerative Colitis journal.

169. You already know about your Ulcerative Colitis symptoms, but learn more about other possible symptoms that may arise in the future.

170. Avoid heavy and long-time exercises during flare-up periods.

171. Try to get enough sleep. Your body needs to rest more than other people do. Sleeping 8 to 9 hours a day (even a little bit more!) would be great.

172. Curcumin is an excellent anti-inflammatory supplement for Ulcerative Colitis patients. Ask your doctor if you want to try curcumin.

173. If you are a long-term Ulcerative Colitis patient, be more aware of the side effects of your drugs. For instance, possible issues such as bone loss (osteoporosis) can develop. Make sure you are getting enough calcium, vitamin-D, and other required nutrients to maintain your health. Check regularly your treatment plan with your doctor.

174. If any Ulcerative Colitis complications caused other serious health issues, you need to consider these issues in your daily life plans fully. Follow the steps your gastroenterologist recommends. In complicated cases, you may need to seek other specialist's opinions.

175. If you are in remission, it is always a great idea to take inflammation blood (C-reactive protein) or stool (Fecal Calprotectin Test) test monthly to see if there is any inflammation in your body and gut that can lead to a flare-up or not.

176. Talk to your doctor about any required endoscopic or imaging procedures you need to follow regularly.

177. If you think you can participate in new clinical studies related to your Ulcerative Colitis disease, talk to your doctor about it first. Take time for your decision and decide with common sense considering different aspects of choosing this decision. Remember that researchers highly appreciate your participation.

178. Avoid consuming artificial sweeteners during flares and remissions.

179. Avoid consuming High Fructose Corn Syrup (HFCS) products all the times.

180. Lemon and lime are generally safe to consume. Always check your tolerance regarding them, especially during flares.

181. Remember that if you are consuming triggering and irritating foods during the remission period, you are more vulnerable to have a flare-up compared to those who do not consume such foods.

182. Do not sit on the toilet for too long. Do not push your stool out much as well, even if you feel that your stomach has not fully emptied.

183. If you had colostomy surgery, make sure you know how to use the Stoma and clean it.

184. If a doctor recommends surgery, always ask the second opinion.

185. If you decided to go for surgery, follow all the necessary steps your doctors recommend.

186. Intravenous (IV) Iron Infusion is one of the great options for Ulcerative Colitis patients who cannot absorb Iron well. Ask your doctor about the IV iron infusion option for you.

187. Be patient with your medications. Many of them need time to be effective. For instance, biologics need a couple of months to be effective.

188. Vitamin B9, B12, D, A, E, & K, Calcium, Folic Acid, Iron, Magnesium, Zinc, and Potassium are some of the typical supplements required for Ulcerative Colitis patients.

189. The calcium supplement is most effective when taken together with vitamin D.

190. Some studies show probiotics benefits to Ulcerative Colitis patients. However, further studies need to check the effectiveness of probiotic types and impact on maintaining remission. Yogurts, kefir, tempeh, miso, and sauerkraut are some of the natural sources of probiotics.

191. Prebiotics are not living bacteria but foods for good bacteria. They are the most customarily digested carbohydrates that can be found in foods such as legumes, fruits, and whole grains. By consuming prebiotics, you can select living bacteria that you want to grow more in your gut.

192. If an Ulcerative Colitis patient consumes steroids such as prednisone in high doses for a long period, or long-lasting diarrhea or blood loss, she/he may need to take protein supplements as well.

193. Increase your knowledge about Ulcerative Colitis by reading books like this and other publications or use other reliable sources. It is always better to rely on scientifically proven sources.

194. Make a great relationship with your doctor. Try to schedule appointments and express your condition with no hesitation to your doctor. List your symptoms, feelings, and any questions you want to ask your doctor. It is not a bad idea to have a close family member or a friend with you during your appointment with your doctor.

195. Provide yourself with Ulcerative Colitis management programs for both flare-up and remission periods.

196. Remember that if you diagnosed with Ulcerative Colitis, it is not your fault. Researches showed Ulcerative Colitis's multifactorial properties. In other words, three main factors

are likely to be involved in Developing Ulcerative Colitis: Genetics, Environment, and Immune System Malfunction.

197. Remember to change any daily habits that can trigger your disease.

198. Understand what to consume and what not to consume step-by-step by using an Ulcerative Colitis journal.

199. Visit emergency in emergency circumstances, such as bleeding a lot or irresistible pains.

200. There are many ongoing research studies related to Ulcerative Colitis disease. Many researchers are devoted to focus on developing new treatments for Ulcerative Colitis patients. Some experts expect that a wave of new treatment solutions is on the way for Ulcerative Colitis patients. So, keep hope tremendously alive!

LAST WORDS...

This book aimed to provide you with useful information about UC healthy nutritional choices, food preparation, how to cook for Ulcerative Colitis patients, and essential dietary steps you need to follow to manage UC effectively. It also guided you through meal planning, how to create biweekly cooking plans.

Comprehensive lists of foods to avoid and foods to each for Ulcerative Colitis patients for flare-up and remission periods presented in Chapter 3, and Chapter 8 suggested essential hints about how to cook for Ulcerative Colitis patients. You learned more than 130 different cooking recipes presented in Chapter 5 of this book, including cooking tips and UC-related tips.

Chapter 6 provided essential tips for Ulcerative Colitis patients food preparation and meal planning. Chapter 7 presented biweekly cooking plan samples for flare-up and remission periods. The blanked biweekly cooking plan tables in this chapter can be used by you to write your own cooking plans. Remember that it is always essential to talk to your doctor about suggested foods or any recommended diets you would like to follow.

Chapter 8 presented the top 200 tips for Ulcerative Colitis patients to live healthier and happier. You can print this chapter to review essential tips for Ulcerative Colitis patients any time you wish.

Now, you have read and learned almost all the basics about UC-related diets, food preparation, and meal plans by reading this book. If you would like to know about another type of Inflammatory Bowel Disease (IBD) called Crohn's disease in detail and how to manage it to have a better lifestyle, you can read the following books in the amazon kindle store written by the same author of this book:

The Comprehensive Guide to Crohn's Disease, All You Need to Know About Crohn's Disease, from Diagnosis to Management & Treatment, by Monet Manbacci, P.h.D., Available in Amazon Kindle and Paperback formats, 2019.

Crohn's Disease Comprehensive Diet Guide and Cookbook, by Monet Manbacci, P.h.D., Available in Amazon Kindle and Paperback formats, 2019.

Moreover, if you found out that you would like to have a comprehensive journal/diary or a calendar that has been designed explicitly for Ulcerative Colitis patients to record all your UC-related history, you may want to take a look at the following book in the amazon store prepared by the same author of this book:

My Ulcerative Colitis Journal, A Comprehensive Planner & Guide for Ulcerative Colitis patients, by Monet Manbacci, P.h.D., Available in Amazon Paperback Format, Dec. 2019.

ONE LAST THING...

The author of this book would like to thank you for reading this book and hope the book was helpful to you.

If you found this book useful or learned something from it, It would be much appreciated if you write a short review on the Amazon website.

The success of such books highly depends on your honest reviews. Your reviews can help the author improve the quality of this book in the next revisions. It can help other people to make informed decisions about reading this book as well.

If you have any feedback, comments or questions, feel free to email Monet Manbacci: monetmanbacci@gmail.com

Thanks again for your support!

ABOUT THE AUTHOR

Monet Manbacci, Ph.D., is the author of *"Ulcerative Colitis Comprehensive Diet Guide and Cookbook"*, *"The Comprehensive Guide to Crohn's Disease"*, and *"Ulcerative Colitis Journal"* Books. He is an IBD patient who has a Doctor of Philosophy (Ph.D.) degree in Applied Sciences and has been involved in academic and scientific research for more than 14 years.

OTHER BOOKS BY HEALTHVIEW PUBLISHERS:

My Ulcerative Colitis Journal, A Comprehensive Planner & Guide for Ulcerative Colitis patients, by Monet Manbacci, P.h.D., Available in Amazon Paperback Format, Dec. 2019.

Crohn's Disease Comprehensive Diet Guide and Cookbook, by Monet Manbacci, P.h.D., Available in Amazon Kindle & Paperback Formats, 2019.

The Comprehensive Guide to Crohn's Disease, All You Need to Know About Crohn's Disease, from Diagnosis to Management & Treatment, by Monet Manbacci, P.h.D., Available in Amazon Kindle & Paperback Formats, 2019.

My Crohn's Disease Journal, A Comprehensive Planner & Guide for Crohn's patients, by Monet Manbacci, P.h.D., Available in Amazon Paperback Format, Dec. 2019.

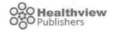

Made in the USA
San Bernardino, CA
07 March 2020

65409443R00197